# AUTOIMMUNE HEPATITIS

## COOKBOOK FOR BEGINNERS

Nourishing Recipes and Practical Tips for Managing Your Health, Supporting Liver Function, and Enhancing Your Well-Being

Kingsley Klopp

**To show our appreciation for your purchase, we're delighted to offer you these special bonuses as a heartfelt thank you**

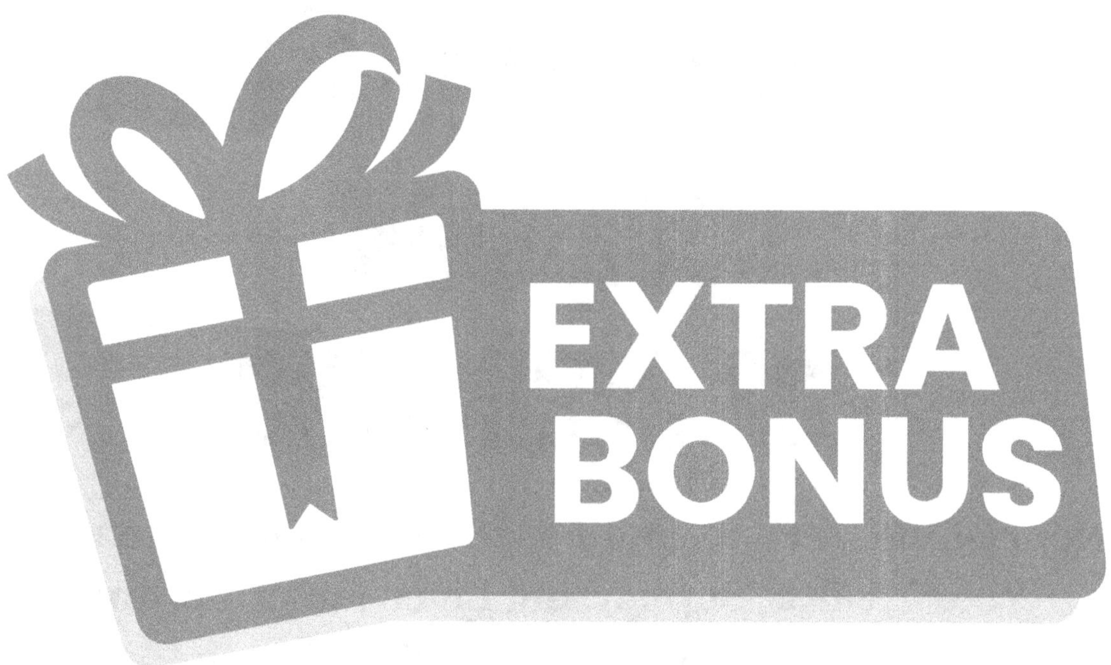


1. A Food Tracker Journal
2. Downloadable E-BOOK featuring full-color images of finished recipes

# Table of Content

# Important Note

This book is crafted with love and care, aimed at guiding you on a journey towards better health through delicious and nourishing meals. However, it's essential to remember that while we strive to provide valuable information and recipes tailored for those managing autoimmune hepatitis, every individual is unique.

Autoimmune hepatitis can manifest differently in each person, and dietary needs may vary widely. The recipes in this cookbook are designed to support liver health and reduce inflammation, but it's crucial to adjust them based on your specific needs and preferences. Listen to your body and make modifications as necessary to ensure that your meals are both enjoyable and beneficial for your condition.

We strongly encourage you to consult with your healthcare provider before making significant changes to your diet. Your doctor or a registered dietitian can offer personalized advice and ensure that the dietary choices you make align with your overall treatment plan. If you ever feel uncertain or have questions about how a particular recipe might affect your health, don't hesitate to seek their guidance.

Additionally, please note that the nutritional information provided in this book is approximate. The values may vary based on the specific ingredients and brands you use, as well as your portion sizes. Consider this information as a general guide to help you make informed choices, but not an exact measure.

Furthermore, If our cookbook has brought joy to your kitchen and table, we'd be thrilled to hear about your experiences in an Amazon review. On the flip side, if you stumble upon any hiccups while exploring our recipes, don't hesitate to get in touch at **kloppkingsley@gmail.com.** We're here to support your cooking journey every step of the way

Our goal is to support and empower you on your health journey, offering recipes that bring joy and nourishment to your table. Cooking and eating should be a delightful experience, and we hope this cookbook helps you discover new flavors and meals that you love.

# *Introduction*

Welcome to **Autoimmune Hepatitis Cookbook for Beginners** – your ultimate guide to nourishing your body and soul while managing autoimmune hepatitis. If you're reading this, chances are you or someone you love has been diagnosed with this chronic liver condition. First and foremost, let me assure you that you are not alone. Millions of people worldwide are navigating this journey, and while it can be challenging, it is also a journey of hope, empowerment, and rediscovery of food. Autoimmune hepatitis can be a daunting diagnosis. The words alone might evoke fear and uncertainty. Questions swirl in your mind: What does this mean for my health? How will this affect my daily life? What can I eat? The good news is that with the right approach, you can manage your condition and still enjoy a rich, flavorful diet. This cookbook is designed to be your companion on this journey, offering delicious, nutritious, and easy-to-prepare recipes that support your liver health and overall well-being.

Food is more than just fuel; it's a fundamental part of our lives. It brings joy, comfort, and connection. When managing a condition like autoimmune hepatitis, the right diet can make a significant difference in how you feel day-to-day. It can help reduce inflammation, support liver function, and boost your immune system. This cookbook is not just about avoiding certain foods; it's about embracing a wide variety of delicious ingredients that are beneficial to your health. Imagine waking up to a vibrant Green Goddess Smoothie, bursting with antioxidants and vitamins that kick-start your day. Picture yourself enjoying a hearty bowl of Chicken and Rice Soup with Lemon for lunch, warming and soothing with every spoonful. And for dinner, how about savoring a Moroccan Vegetable Stew with Chickpeas, rich in flavor and nutrients? These are just a few examples of the culinary delights awaiting you in these pages. We understand that starting a new diet can be overwhelming, especially when dealing with a medical condition. That's why this cookbook is tailored specifically for beginners. You don't need to be a seasoned chef to whip up these meals. Each recipe is crafted with simplicity in mind, featuring step-by-step instructions, accessible ingredients, and practical tips to make your cooking experience enjoyable and stress-free. Whether you're cooking for yourself, your family, or friends, these recipes are designed to fit into your busy life without compromising on taste or nutrition.

But this book is more than just a collection of recipes. It's a resource packed with valuable information about autoimmune hepatitis and the role of diet in managing this condition. You'll find sections dedicated to understanding the basics of autoimmune hepatitis, the importance of a liver-friendly diet, and practical advice on shopping for and preparing meals that support your health. We delve into the science behind anti-inflammatory foods and why certain ingredients are particularly beneficial for those with autoimmune hepatitis. In addition to the recipes, you'll also discover meal planning tips to help you stay organized and consistent with your dietary choices. The comprehensive 10-week meal plan provided in this book takes the guesswork out of what to eat, offering a structured yet flexible approach to meal planning that ensures you get a balanced intake of nutrients every day.

We know that every individual's journey with autoimmune hepatitis is unique. That's why the recipes in this book are easily adaptable to suit your personal tastes and dietary needs. Feel free to experiment with different ingredients and make these dishes your own. The goal is to empower you to take control of your health through the food you eat, transforming your kitchen into a place of healing and enjoyment. Setting out on this dietary journey might seem challenging at first, but remember, you are capable of making positive changes. With each meal you prepare, you're taking a step towards better health and well-being. This cookbook is here to support you every step of the way, offering guidance, inspiration, and delicious recipes that make eating for autoimmune hepatitis a pleasure, not a chore.

So, let's get started. Open your pantry, fire up your stove, and embrace the joy of cooking with "Autoimmune Hepatitis Cookbook for Beginners." Your journey to better health begins here, one delicious meal at a time. Welcome to a world of flavorful, nourishing food that loves your liver as much as you do.

# Chapter 1: Understanding Autoimmune Hepatitis

## *What is Autoimmune Hepatitis?*

Autoimmune Hepatitis (AIH) is a chronic and often relentless liver disease that, despite its complexity and seriousness, remains a topic shrouded in mystery for many. Imagine the body's immune system, typically our guardian against infections and diseases, suddenly misidentifying its own liver cells as foreign invaders. This misidentification prompts the immune system to launch a misguided attack on the liver, causing inflammation and damage over time. This is the essence of Autoimmune Hepatitis – a condition where the body's defense mechanism turns against itself, leading to potentially devastating consequences. To truly grasp the impact of AIH, one must first understand the profound role of the liver in our bodies. The liver is an extraordinary organ, tirelessly working to detoxify the blood, produce vital proteins, aid in digestion, and store nutrients that our bodies depend on for energy. When the liver is under attack, every aspect of our health can be affected, making AIH a disease that goes beyond the confines of the liver.

For those diagnosed with AIH, the journey often begins with a sense of confusion and fear. Unlike more well-known conditions, AIH does not always come with a clear set of triggers or causes. It can strike at any age and affects women more frequently than men. The exact reasons why the immune system turns against the liver are still being researched, but it is believed that a combination of genetic predisposition and environmental factors, such as infections or toxins, may play a role. This uncertainty can be daunting for patients and their families, who are left wondering why this has happened to them. Living with AIH is akin to walking a tightrope. The disease can be unpredictable, with periods of relative calm interrupted by sudden flare-ups, where symptoms intensify, and liver damage can accelerate. These flare-ups can be physically and emotionally exhausting, as individuals must constantly monitor their health and be vigilant about any changes in their condition. The emotional toll of living with a chronic illness cannot be overstated. Patients often grapple with feelings of frustration, anxiety, and isolation, as they navigate a condition that many around them may not fully understand.

One of the most challenging aspects of AIH is its impact on daily life. Fatigue is a common and debilitating symptom, making even the simplest tasks feel insurmountable. This persistent tiredness is not just about feeling sleepy; it is a deep, unrelenting exhaustion that can drain the joy out of everyday activities. Imagine waking up each day feeling as though you have not slept at all, struggling to find the energy to go to work, care for your family, or even enjoy your hobbies. This fatigue can lead to a significant reduction in quality of life, affecting mental health and overall well-being. Moreover, dietary changes are often necessary for managing AIH, adding another layer of complexity to daily routines. Patients must be mindful of what they eat, avoiding certain foods that may exacerbate liver inflammation. This can mean a complete overhaul of eating habits, which can be both challenging and frustrating. Social activities that revolve around food, such as dining out with friends or family gatherings, can become sources of stress and anxiety. The need to constantly explain dietary restrictions can make individuals feel like outsiders in their own lives.

The social implications of AIH are profound. Living with a chronic illness can strain relationships, as loved ones may struggle to understand the invisible nature of the disease. The lack of outward symptoms can lead to misunderstandings, with others questioning the severity of the condition or assuming that the person is simply not trying hard enough to stay healthy. This lack of understanding can result in a sense of isolation, where patients feel alone in their battle against AIH. Despite these challenges, there is hope. Advances in medical research are providing new insights into the mechanisms of AIH, paving the way for better treatments and, ultimately, a cure. Support groups and communities, both online and offline, offer a lifeline to those affected, providing a space to share experiences, find support, and draw strength from others who understand the journey.

Autoimmune Hepatitis is a complex and demanding condition, but it is one that can be managed with the right knowledge, support, and care. Understanding AIH is the first step in combating it. For those diagnosed, it is crucial to remember that they are not alone, and that there are resources and communities ready to offer support. Embracing the journey with resilience and hope can make all the difference in living a fulfilling life despite the challenges posed by Autoimmune Hepatitis.

# Symptoms and Diagnosis

**Symptoms of Autoimmune Hepatitis**

Autoimmune Hepatitis (AIH) manifests with a range of symptoms that can vary greatly from person to person. These symptoms often reflect the liver's central role in the body, and the inflammation caused by AIH can disrupt many of its vital functions. Understanding these symptoms is crucial for recognizing the disease early and seeking appropriate medical care.

1. Fatigue
   - One of the most common and debilitating symptoms of AIH is fatigue. This is not just ordinary tiredness but a profound, unrelenting exhaustion that doesn't improve with rest. It can severely impact daily life, making even simple tasks feel overwhelming.
2. Jaundice
   - Jaundice is characterized by a yellowing of the skin and the whites of the eyes. This occurs due to the buildup of bilirubin, a yellow pigment that the liver usually processes and eliminates. When the liver is inflamed and not functioning properly, bilirubin can accumulate in the blood.
3. Abdominal Discomfort
   - Patients often experience pain or discomfort in the upper right quadrant of the abdomen, where the liver is located. This can range from a dull ache to more severe pain, depending on the extent of liver inflammation.
4. Joint Pain
   - AIH can also cause joint pain and swelling, often affecting the small joints of the hands and feet. This symptom can sometimes be mistaken for other autoimmune conditions, such as rheumatoid arthritis.
5. Skin Manifestations
   - Some individuals with AIH may develop skin conditions, such as rashes, acne, or the appearance of spider angiomas (small, spider-like blood vessels visible under the skin).
6. Nausea and Loss of Appetite
   - Inflammation of the liver can lead to gastrointestinal symptoms, including nausea, vomiting, and a loss of appetite. This can result in unintended weight loss and nutritional deficiencies.
7. Dark Urine and Pale Stools
   - As bilirubin levels rise, it can cause urine to become dark and stools to become pale. This is a direct result of the liver's impaired ability to process and excrete bilirubin.
8. Fever and Malaise
   - Some patients may experience general malaise, fever, and flu-like symptoms, which can be mistaken for a viral infection initially.

**Diagnosis of Autoimmune Hepatitis**

Diagnosing Autoimmune Hepatitis can be challenging due to the variability of symptoms and their overlap with other liver and autoimmune diseases. A comprehensive diagnostic process typically involves a combination of medical history, physical examination, blood tests, imaging studies, and sometimes a liver biopsy.

1. Medical History and Physical Examination
   - The diagnostic journey begins with a thorough medical history, including any family history of autoimmune diseases, and a detailed account of symptoms. A physical examination may reveal signs of liver disease, such as jaundice or an enlarged liver.

2. Blood Tests
   - Liver Function Tests (LFTs): These tests measure levels of liver enzymes (ALT, AST, ALP) and bilirubin in the blood. Elevated levels indicate liver inflammation or damage.
   - Autoantibody Tests: Specific autoantibodies are often present in AIH. Common ones include anti-nuclear antibodies (ANA), anti-smooth muscle antibodies (ASMA), and liver/kidney microsomal antibodies (LKM-1). Their presence helps support the diagnosis.
   - IgG Levels: Elevated levels of immunoglobulin G (IgG) can also suggest AIH, as they indicate increased immune activity.

3. Imaging Studies
   - Imaging tests such as ultrasound, CT scans, or MRI may be used to evaluate the liver's size, shape, and texture, as well as to rule out other conditions such as tumors or bile duct obstructions.

4. Liver Biopsy
   - A liver biopsy involves taking a small tissue sample from the liver for microscopic examination. This procedure is often crucial for confirming the diagnosis of AIH. It can reveal the extent of liver inflammation, fibrosis (scarring), and characteristic histological features of AIH, such as interface hepatitis.

5. Exclusion of Other Conditions
   - Since AIH symptoms overlap with those of other liver diseases (e.g., viral hepatitis, alcoholic liver disease, non-alcoholic fatty liver disease), it is essential to rule out these conditions through additional testing, including viral hepatitis panels and assessments of alcohol consumption.

The process of diagnosing AIH can be lengthy and requires patience and collaboration between the patient and healthcare providers. Early and accurate diagnosis is vital for managing the disease effectively and preventing long-term liver damage.

# *Treatment and Management of Autoimmune Hepatitis*

## Medications for Autoimmune Hepatitis

1. Corticosteroids
   - The cornerstone of AIH treatment is corticosteroids, such as prednisone or prednisolone. These medications are powerful anti-inflammatory agents that help reduce the immune system's attack on the liver. Typically, a high dose is prescribed initially to bring the disease under control, followed by a gradual tapering to the lowest effective dose to maintain remission while minimizing side effects. Long-term use of corticosteroids can have significant side effects, including weight gain, osteoporosis, diabetes, and increased infection risk, so careful monitoring is essential.

2. Immunosuppressants
   - In addition to corticosteroids, other immunosuppressive drugs are often used to help control AIH. Azathioprine is the most commonly prescribed immunosuppressant. It works by reducing the activity of the immune system, thereby decreasing liver inflammation. Azathioprine can take several weeks to become effective, so it is often used in conjunction with corticosteroids initially. Other immunosuppressants, such as mycophenolate mofetil, tacrolimus, or cyclosporine, may be used in cases where azathioprine is not tolerated or is ineffective.

3. Combination Therapy
   - Many patients require a combination of corticosteroids and immunosuppressants to achieve and maintain remission. The combination allows for lower doses of each medication, potentially reducing the risk of side effects while effectively controlling the disease.

4. Maintenance Therapy
   - Once remission is achieved, long-term maintenance therapy is necessary to prevent relapse. This often involves continued use of low-dose corticosteroids or immunosuppressants. Some patients may eventually be able to taper off medications entirely, but this decision must be made cautiously and under strict medical supervision.

## Lifestyle Adjustments

1. Diet and Nutrition
   - A healthy diet is crucial for managing AIH and supporting liver health. Patients are advised to eat a balanced diet rich in fruits, vegetables, lean proteins, and whole grains while avoiding foods that can exacerbate liver inflammation, such as high-fat, high-sugar, and highly processed foods. Alcohol should be avoided entirely, as it can significantly worsen liver damage.
2. Exercise
   - Regular physical activity helps maintain overall health, reduces stress, and supports weight management. However, patients should consult their healthcare provider before starting any new exercise regimen, especially during periods of active disease.
3. Avoiding Toxins
   - Patients with AIH should avoid exposure to environmental toxins and medications that can harm the liver. This includes over-the-counter medications, herbal supplements, and certain prescription drugs. Always consult a healthcare provider before taking any new medication or supplement.

## Regular Monitoring and Medical Follow-Up

1. Liver Function Tests
   - Regular blood tests to monitor liver function are essential for managing AIH. These tests help assess the effectiveness of treatment and detect any signs of liver damage or relapse early.
2. Imaging Studies
   - Periodic imaging studies, such as ultrasound, CT scans, or MRI, may be necessary to monitor liver health and detect complications such as cirrhosis or liver cancer.
3. Liver Biopsies
   - Repeat liver biopsies may be required in some cases to assess the degree of liver inflammation and fibrosis, especially if there is a change in symptoms or a concern about disease progression.
4. Specialist Care
   - Management of AIH typically requires ongoing care from a hepatologist (liver specialist) or a gastroenterologist. These specialists have the expertise to tailor treatment plans, adjust medications, and monitor for potential complications.

**Emotional and Psychological Support**
1. Mental Health
   - Living with a chronic illness like AIH can take a significant emotional toll. Patients may experience anxiety, depression, or stress related to their condition. Access to mental health support, such as counseling or therapy, can be beneficial.
2. Support Groups
   - Joining a support group for individuals with AIH or other chronic liver diseases can provide emotional support, practical advice, and a sense of community. Sharing experiences with others who understand the challenges of living with AIH can be incredibly reassuring and empowering.

Managing Complications
1. Cirrhosis
   - In cases where AIH has led to cirrhosis, additional medical management is necessary to address complications such as portal hypertension, varices, and liver failure. This may involve medications, lifestyle changes, and sometimes surgical interventions.
2. Liver Transplant
   - In severe cases where the liver has sustained significant damage and medical therapy is no longer effective, a liver transplant may be considered. This is a complex procedure that involves replacing the diseased liver with a healthy one from a donor. Post-transplant, patients require lifelong immunosuppressive therapy to prevent organ rejection.

# Chapter 2: The Role of Diet in Autoimmune Hepatitis

## *Anti-inflammatory Foods*

The role of diet in managing Autoimmune Hepatitis (AIH) is critical, particularly when it comes to incorporating anti-inflammatory foods into daily meals. Chronic inflammation is a hallmark of AIH, where the immune system erroneously attacks the liver, leading to ongoing liver inflammation and damage. Therefore, adopting a diet rich in anti-inflammatory foods can help mitigate this inflammation, support liver health, and enhance overall well-being. Anti-inflammatory foods are those that can help reduce inflammation in the body. These foods contain various compounds, such as antioxidants, polyphenols, omega-3 fatty acids, and other bioactive substances, that combat oxidative stress and inflammatory processes. Incorporating these foods into your diet can play a crucial role in managing AIH by potentially reducing liver inflammation and promoting a healthier immune response.

**Key Anti-inflammatory Foods**

1. Fatty Fish
   - Fatty fish such as salmon, mackerel, sardines, and trout are rich in omega-3 fatty acids. These essential fats, specifically EPA and DHA, have potent anti-inflammatory properties. Omega-3 fatty acids help decrease the production of inflammatory molecules and cytokines, which are substances secreted by immune cells that can contribute to inflammation. Regular consumption of fatty fish can support liver health and reduce the overall inflammatory burden on the body.

2. Leafy Green Vegetables
   - Leafy greens like spinach, kale, Swiss chard, and collard greens are packed with vitamins, minerals, and antioxidants. They are particularly rich in vitamin K, which has been shown to have anti-inflammatory effects. These vegetables also contain high levels of polyphenols and fiber, both of which help lower inflammation and improve gut health.

3. Berries
- Berries such as blueberries, strawberries, raspberries, and blackberries are among the best sources of antioxidants, including vitamin C and various polyphenols. These compounds help neutralize free radicals, reducing oxidative stress and inflammation. The fiber content in berries also supports a healthy digestive system, which is important for overall health and well-being.

4. Nuts and Seeds
- Nuts like almonds, walnuts, and seeds such as chia seeds, flaxseeds, and hemp seeds are excellent sources of healthy fats, fiber, and protein. They are also rich in omega-3 fatty acids, particularly walnuts and flaxseeds, which can help reduce inflammation. Additionally, nuts and seeds contain antioxidants and other bioactive compounds that support immune function and reduce inflammatory responses.

5. Olive Oil
- Extra virgin olive oil is a staple of the Mediterranean diet, known for its numerous health benefits, including its anti-inflammatory properties. It is rich in monounsaturated fats and antioxidants, particularly oleocanthal, which has been shown to have similar effects to anti-inflammatory drugs like ibuprofen. Incorporating olive oil into your diet can help reduce liver inflammation and promote heart health.

6. Turmeric
- Turmeric is a vibrant yellow spice commonly used in Indian cuisine. Its active ingredient, curcumin, has powerful anti-inflammatory and antioxidant properties. Curcumin helps inhibit inflammatory pathways in the body, making turmeric a valuable addition to an anti-inflammatory diet. Pairing turmeric with black pepper enhances the absorption of curcumin, making it even more effective.

7. Ginger
- Ginger is another spice with potent anti-inflammatory effects. It contains bioactive compounds like gingerol and shogaol, which help reduce inflammation and oxidative stress. Ginger can be used in various forms, including fresh, dried, or as a tea, to help support liver health and overall inflammation management.

8. Garlic
- Garlic is renowned for its health benefits, including its anti-inflammatory properties. It contains sulfur compounds that help inhibit inflammatory enzymes and reduce the production of inflammatory molecules. Adding garlic to your meals can provide flavor and health benefits, supporting a balanced and anti-inflammatory diet.

9. Green Tea
  - Green tea is rich in polyphenols, particularly catechins, which have strong anti-inflammatory and antioxidant effects. Regular consumption of green tea can help reduce inflammation, support liver health, and provide a soothing, healthy beverage option.
10. Whole Grains
  - Whole grains such as brown rice, quinoa, oats, and barley are high in fiber and various nutrients that support overall health. Unlike refined grains, whole grains have anti-inflammatory properties due to their high fiber content, which helps regulate blood sugar levels and promotes a healthy gut microbiome.

# *Foods to Avoid*

Managing Autoimmune Hepatitis (AIH) involves not only incorporating anti-inflammatory foods into your diet but also being vigilant about avoiding certain foods that can exacerbate liver inflammation and damage. The liver is crucial for detoxifying the body, processing nutrients, and maintaining overall health. When it is compromised by AIH, consuming foods that strain or damage the liver can lead to more severe health issues. Here's a comprehensive look at the foods to avoid for better management of AIH.

1. Alcohol
- Why Avoid? Alcohol is particularly harmful to the liver, even in small amounts. It increases inflammation and accelerates liver damage, leading to conditions like fatty liver disease, cirrhosis, and liver failure.
- Impact on AIH: Alcohol can worsen the symptoms of AIH and interfere with the effectiveness of medications used to manage the condition. It can also increase the risk of developing liver cancer.
- Alternative: Opt for non-alcoholic beverages like herbal teas, infused water, or sparkling water with a splash of natural fruit juice.

2. High-Fat Foods
- Why Avoid? Foods high in saturated and trans fats can contribute to fatty liver disease, which complicates the management of AIH. These fats can increase cholesterol levels and promote inflammation.
- Common Sources: Fried foods, fast food, processed snacks, pastries, and fatty cuts of meat.
- Impact on AIH: High-fat foods can exacerbate liver inflammation and impair liver function.
- Alternative: Choose healthy fats such as those found in avocados, nuts, seeds, and fatty fish. Cook with olive oil or other healthy oils instead of butter or lard.

3. Sugary Foods and Beverages
- Why Avoid? Excessive sugar intake can lead to insulin resistance, obesity, and non-alcoholic fatty liver disease (NAFLD), all of which strain the liver.
- Common Sources: Sodas, candies, baked goods, and sugary cereals.
- Impact on AIH: High sugar consumption can worsen liver inflammation and overall health, making it harder to manage AIH.
- Alternative: Use natural sweeteners like honey or maple syrup in moderation. Incorporate whole fruits instead of sugary snacks to satisfy sweet cravings.

4. Refined Carbohydrates
- Why Avoid? Refined carbs, such as white bread, pasta, and pastries, have a high glycemic index, leading to rapid spikes in blood sugar and increased fat storage in the liver.
- Impact on AIH: These foods can contribute to insulin resistance and liver inflammation, complicating the management of AIH.
- Alternative: Choose whole grains like brown rice, quinoa, whole-wheat bread, and oats, which provide fiber and nutrients without spiking blood sugar levels.

5. Processed and Preserved Foods
- Why Avoid? Processed foods often contain unhealthy additives, preservatives, and high levels of sodium and sugar. These can burden the liver and increase inflammation.
- Common Sources: Processed meats (sausages, hot dogs, deli meats), canned soups, and ready-to-eat meals.
- Impact on AIH: The additives and preservatives can exacerbate liver inflammation and interfere with liver function.
- Alternative: Opt for fresh, whole foods and prepare meals at home to control ingredients. If using canned or preserved foods, choose options with low sodium and no added sugars or preservatives.

6. High-Sodium Foods
- Why Avoid? Excessive sodium intake can lead to fluid retention and high blood pressure, putting additional stress on the liver and cardiovascular system.
- Common Sources: Salted snacks, processed foods, canned soups, and fast food.
- Impact on AIH: High sodium levels can worsen liver function and contribute to fluid buildup in the abdomen (ascites), a common complication in liver disease.
- Alternative: Use herbs and spices to flavor foods instead of salt. Choose low-sodium or no-salt-added versions of canned and processed foods.

7. Red and Processed Meats
- Why Avoid? Red meats and processed meats are high in saturated fats and cholesterol, which can promote liver inflammation and damage.
- Common Sources: Beef, pork, lamb, bacon, sausages, and deli meats.
- Impact on AIH: These meats can increase the risk of fatty liver disease and exacerbate liver inflammation.
- Alternative: Choose lean protein sources such as chicken, turkey, fish, legumes, and plant-based proteins like tofu and tempeh.

8. Dairy Products
- Why Avoid? Full-fat dairy products can be high in saturated fats, contributing to liver inflammation and fat accumulation.
- Common Sources: Whole milk, cheese, butter, and cream.
- Impact on AIH: High-fat dairy can worsen liver inflammation and overall liver health.
- Alternative: Opt for low-fat or fat-free dairy products, or choose plant-based alternatives like almond milk, soy milk, and coconut yogurt.

9. Artificial Sweeteners and Additives
- Why Avoid? Artificial sweeteners and food additives can burden the liver with additional substances to detoxify, potentially leading to liver stress and inflammation.
- Common Sources: Diet sodas, sugar-free candies, and many processed foods.
- Impact on AIH: These additives can interfere with liver function and exacerbate symptoms of AIH.
- Alternative: Use natural sweeteners like stevia or monk fruit in moderation, and read labels to avoid products with unnecessary additives.

# Breakfast Recipes

## 1. Green Goddess Smoothie

**Ingredients**

- 1 cup fresh spinach
- 1/2 avocado
- 1 banana
- 1/2 cup cucumber, chopped
- 1/2 cup unsweetened almond milk
- 1 tablespoon chia seeds
- Juice of 1/2 lemon
- 1 teaspoon honey (optional)
- Ice cubes (optional)

**Instructions**

1. Add spinach, avocado, banana, cucumber, almond milk, chia seeds, lemon juice, and honey (if using) to a blender.
2. Blend until smooth. If the smoothie is too thick, add a bit more almond milk.
3. Add ice cubes if desired and blend again until smooth.
4. Pour into a glass and enjoy immediately.

**Nutrition Info per Serving**

- Calories: 250
- Protein: 4g
- Carbohydrates: 34g
- Fiber: 9g
- Sugars: 15g
- Fat: 13g
- Saturated Fat: 2g
- Sodium: 70mg

**Servings: 1**
**Cooking Time: 5 minutes**

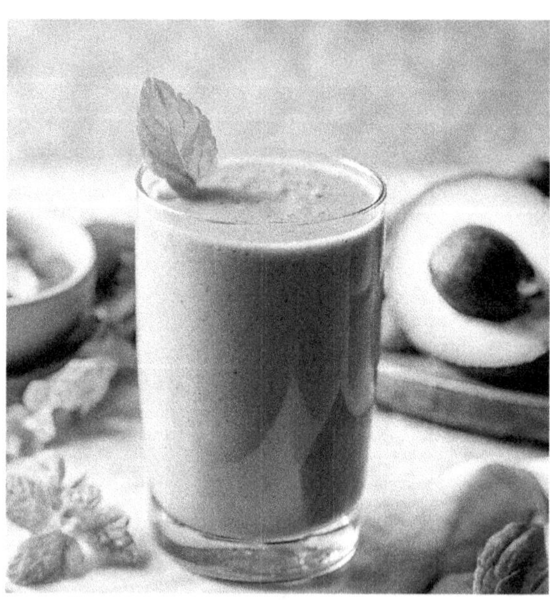

## 2. Turmeric Pineapple Smoothie

**Ingredients**

- 1 cup fresh pineapple chunks
- 1 banana
- 1/2 teaspoon ground turmeric
- 1/2 teaspoon ground ginger
- 1/2 cup unsweetened coconut milk
- 1 tablespoon flaxseeds
- Juice of 1/2 lime
- Ice cubes (optional)

**Instructions**

1. Add pineapple, banana, turmeric, ginger, coconut milk, flaxseeds, and lime juice to a blender.
2. Blend until smooth. If the smoothie is too thick, add a bit more coconut milk.
3. Add ice cubes if desired and blend again until smooth.
4. Pour into a glass and enjoy immediately.

**Nutrition Info per Serving**

- Calories: 220
- Protein: 3g
- Carbohydrates: 46g
- Fiber: 7g
- Sugars: 30g
- Fat: 5g
- Saturated Fat: 3g
- Sodium: 40mg

**Servings: 1**
**Cooking Time: 5 minutes**

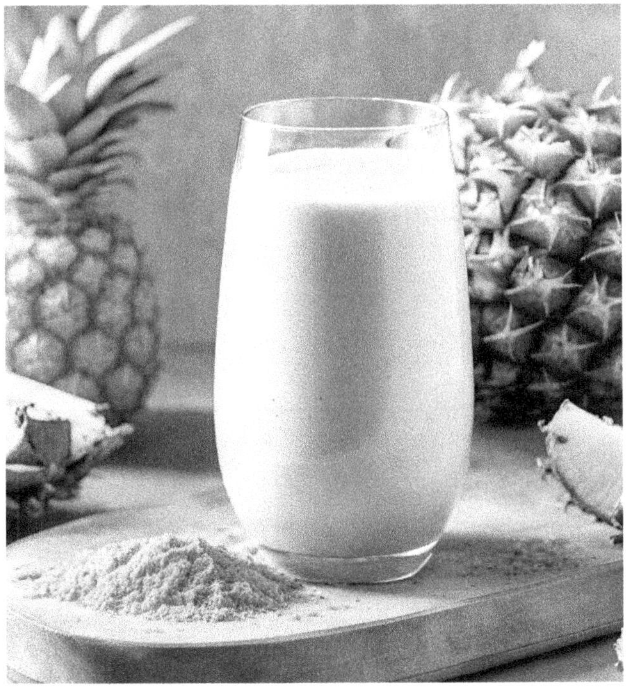

## 3. Apple Cinnamon Porridge

**Ingredients**

- 1/2 cup rolled oats
- 1 cup water or unsweetened almond milk
- 1 apple, peeled, cored, and chopped
- 1/2 teaspoon ground cinnamon
- 1 tablespoon chia seeds
- 1 teaspoon honey (optional)
- 1/4 cup chopped walnuts

**Instructions**

1. In a small pot, combine oats and water or almond milk. Bring to a boil.
2. Reduce heat to a simmer and add chopped apple, cinnamon, and chia seeds. Stir well.
3. Cook for 5-7 minutes, stirring occasionally, until the oats are soft and the mixture has thickened.
4. Remove from heat and stir in honey if using.
5. Pour into a bowl and top with chopped walnuts.
6. Serve warm and enjoy.

**Nutrition Info per Serving**

- Calories: 350
- Protein: 7g
- Carbohydrates: 60g
- Fiber: 10g
- Sugars: 15g
- Fat: 11g
- Saturated Fat: 1g
- Sodium: 10mg

**Servings: 1**
**Cooking Time: 10 minutes**

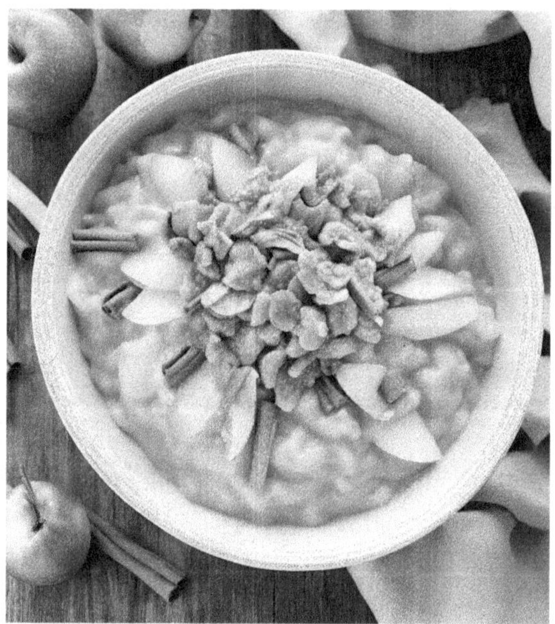

## 4. Savory Oatmeal

### Ingredients

- 1/2 cup rolled oats
- 1 cup water or unsweetened almond milk
- 1/4 cup cherry tomatoes, halved
- 1/4 cup baby spinach
- 1 tablespoon nutritional yeast
- 1 teaspoon olive oil
- 1 poached egg (optional)
- 1/2 teaspoon ground black pepper

### Instructions

1. In a small pot, combine oats and water or almond milk. Bring to a boil.
2. Reduce heat to a simmer and add cherry tomatoes and baby spinach. Stir well.
3. Cook for 5-7 minutes, stirring occasionally, until the oats are soft and the mixture has thickened.
4. Stir in nutritional yeast and olive oil.
5. Transfer to a bowl and top with a poached egg if using.
6. Sprinkle with ground black pepper.
7. Serve warm and enjoy.

### Nutrition Info per Serving (with poached egg)

- Calories: 320
- Protein: 14g
- Carbohydrates: 35g
- Fiber: 7g
- Sugars: 3g
- Fat: 14g
- Saturated Fat: 3g
- Sodium: 100mg

**Servings: 1**

**Cooking Time: 10 minutes**

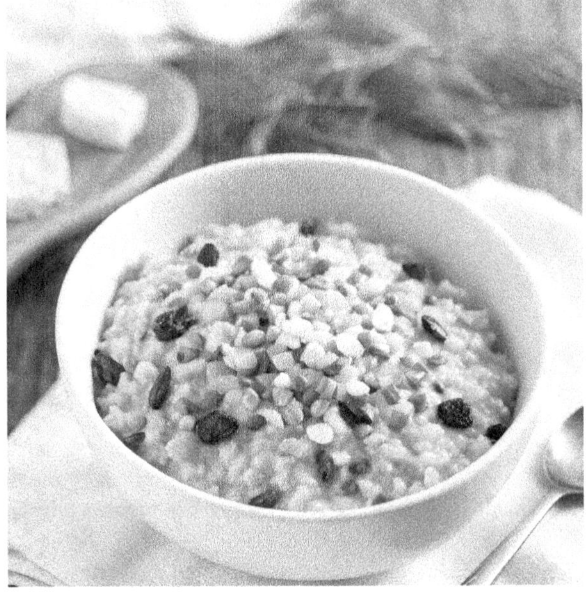

## 5. Scrambled Eggs with Spinach

### Ingredients

- 2 large eggs
- 1 cup fresh baby spinach
- 1 tablespoon olive oil
- 1/4 teaspoon garlic powder
- 1/4 teaspoon onion powder
- 1 tablespoon unsweetened almond milk

### Instructions

1. In a bowl, whisk together the eggs and almond milk until well combined.
2. Heat olive oil in a non-stick skillet over medium heat.
3. Add spinach and cook until wilted, about 2 minutes.
4. Pour the egg mixture into the skillet and add garlic powder and onion powder.
5. Cook, stirring gently, until the eggs are fully cooked but still soft, about 3-4 minutes.
6. Remove from heat and serve immediately.

### Nutrition Info per Serving

- Calories: 200
- Protein: 12g
- Carbohydrates: 3g
- Fiber: 1g
- Sugars: 0g
- Fat: 16g
- Saturated Fat: 3g
- Sodium: 100mg

**Servings: 1**
**Cooking Time: 10 minutes**

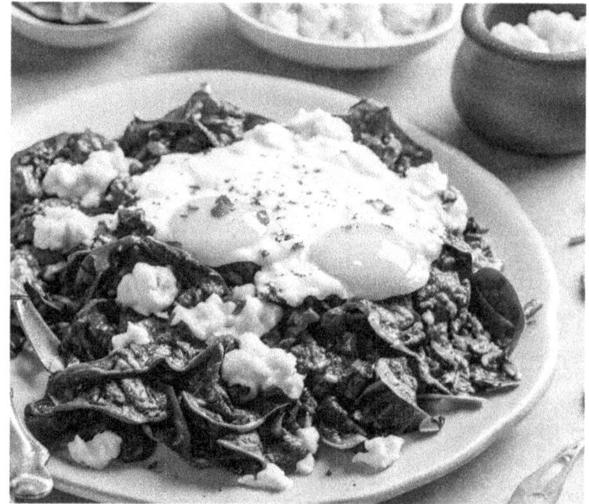

## 6. Omelet with Mixed Veggies

### Ingredients

- 2 large eggs
- 1/4 cup diced bell peppers (any color)
- 1/4 cup diced tomatoes
- 1/4 cup chopped mushrooms
- 1 tablespoon olive oil
- 1/4 teaspoon garlic powder
- 1/4 teaspoon dried oregano
- 1 tablespoon water

### Instructions

1. In a bowl, whisk together the eggs and water until well combined.
2. Heat olive oil in a non-stick skillet over medium heat.
3. Add bell peppers, tomatoes, and mushrooms to the skillet. Cook until vegetables are tender, about 4-5 minutes.
4. Pour the egg mixture over the vegetables and add garlic powder and oregano.
5. Cook without stirring until the eggs begin to set around the edges, about 2-3 minutes.
6. Gently lift the edges of the omelet with a spatula and tilt the skillet to allow uncooked eggs to flow to the edges.
7. Continue cooking until the eggs are fully set, about 2 more minutes.
8. Fold the omelet in half and slide onto a plate. Serve immediately.

### Nutrition Info per Serving

- Calories: 220
- Protein: 12g
- Carbohydrates: 7g
- Fiber: 2g
- Sugars: 3g
- Fat: 16g
- Saturated Fat: 3g
- Sodium: 120mg

**Servings: 1**
**Cooking Time: 15 minutes**

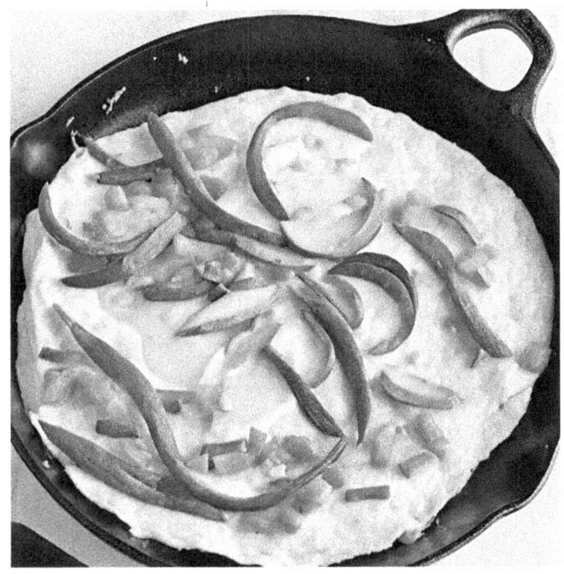

## 7. Tofu Scramble

**Ingredients**

- 1/2 block firm tofu, drained and crumbled
- 1 tablespoon olive oil
- 1/4 cup diced bell peppers (any color)
- 1/4 cup diced tomatoes
- 1/4 cup chopped spinach
- 1/2 teaspoon ground turmeric
- 1/4 teaspoon garlic powder
- 1/4 teaspoon onion powder
- 1 tablespoon nutritional yeast

**Instructions**

1. Heat olive oil in a non-stick skillet over medium heat.
2. Add bell peppers and tomatoes to the skillet. Cook until vegetables are tender, about 3-4 minutes.
3. Add crumbled tofu, spinach, turmeric, garlic powder, and onion powder. Stir well to combine.
4. Cook, stirring occasionally, until the tofu is heated through and the spinach is wilted, about 5-7 minutes.
5. Stir in nutritional yeast and cook for an additional 1 minute.
6. Remove from heat and serve immediately.

**Nutrition Info per Serving**

- Calories: 180
- Protein: 13g
- Carbohydrates: 7g
- Fiber: 3g
- Sugars: 2g
- Fat: 12g
- Saturated Fat: 2g
- Sodium: 120mg

**Servings: 2**
**Cooking Time: 15 minutes**

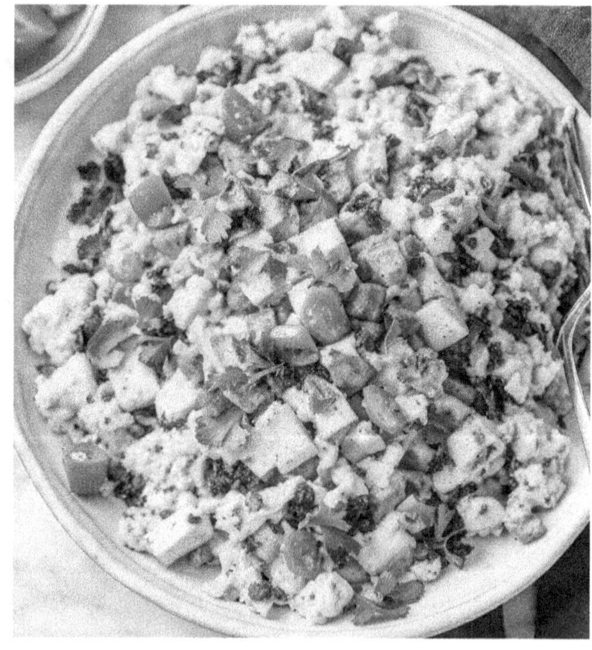

**8. Egg Muffins**
**Ingredients**

- 6 large eggs
- 1/2 cup diced bell peppers (any color)
- 1/2 cup chopped spinach
- 1/4 cup diced onions
- 1/4 cup chopped mushrooms
- 1/4 teaspoon garlic powder
- 1/4 teaspoon dried basil
- 1/4 teaspoon dried oregano
- 1/4 cup unsweetened almond milk
- 1 tablespoon olive oil

**Instructions**

1. Preheat the oven to 350°F (175°C). Grease a muffin tin with olive oil.
2. In a large bowl, whisk together the eggs and almond milk until well combined.
3. Add bell peppers, spinach, onions, mushrooms, garlic powder, basil, and oregano to the egg mixture. Stir well to combine.
4. Pour the mixture evenly into the prepared muffin tin cups.
5. Bake for 20-25 minutes, or until the eggs are set and the tops are golden brown.
6. Remove from the oven and let cool for a few minutes before removing the muffins from the tin.
7. Serve warm or at room temperature.

**Nutrition Info per Serving (2 muffins)**

- Calories: 140
- Protein: 10g
- Carbohydrates: 3g
- Fiber: 1g
- Sugars: 1g
- Fat: 10g
- Saturated Fat: 2g
- Sodium: 100mg

**Servings: 6 muffins (3 servings)**
**Cooking Time: 30 minutes**

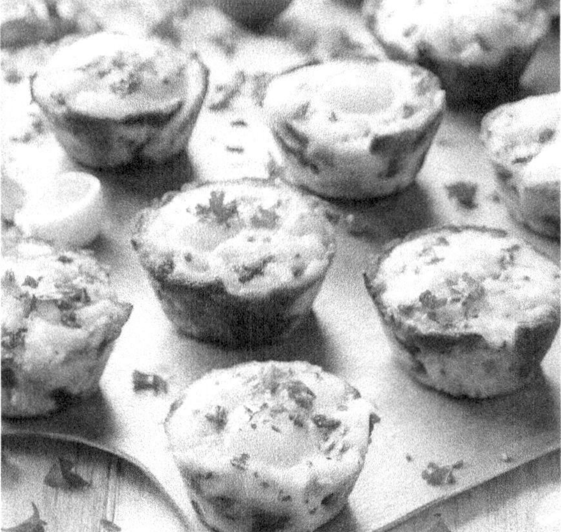

## 9. Ricotta and Berry Toast

**Ingredients**

- 2 slices whole-grain bread
- 1/2 cup ricotta cheese
- 1/2 cup mixed berries (strawberries, blueberries, raspberries)
- 1 teaspoon honey
- 1/4 teaspoon ground cinnamon

**Instructions**

1. Toast the whole-grain bread slices until golden brown.
2. Spread ricotta cheese evenly over each slice of toast.
3. Top with mixed berries.
4. Drizzle honey over the berries.
5. Sprinkle ground cinnamon on top.
6. Serve immediately.

**Nutrition Info per Serving**

- Calories: 220
- Protein: 10g
- Carbohydrates: 32g
- Fiber: 5g
- Sugars: 10g
- Fat: 6g
- Saturated Fat: 3g
- Sodium: 150mg

**Servings: 2**
**Cooking Time: 5 minutes**

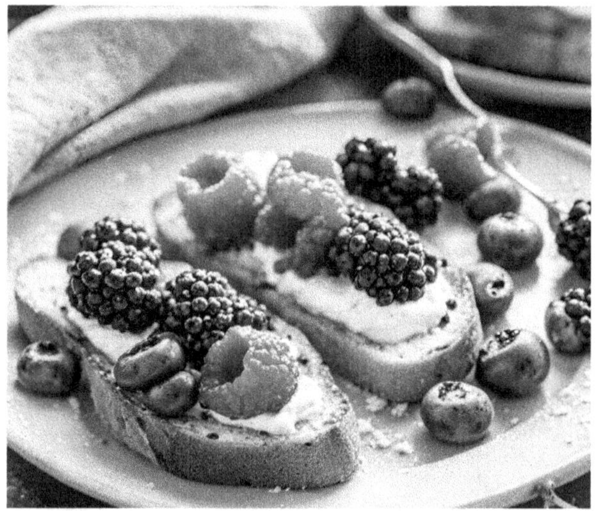

**10. Tahini and Honey Toast**

**Ingredients**

- 2 slices whole-grain bread
- 2 tablespoons tahini
- 1 tablespoon honey
- 1/4 teaspoon ground cinnamon
- 1/4 cup sliced bananas (optional)

**Instructions**

1. Toast the whole-grain bread slices until golden brown.
2. Spread tahini evenly over each slice of toast.
3. Drizzle honey over the tahini.
4. Sprinkle ground cinnamon on top.
5. Optional: Add sliced bananas on top of the toast.
6. Serve immediately.

**Nutrition Info per Serving**

- Calories: 240
- Protein: 7g
- Carbohydrates: 34g
- Fiber: 5g
- Sugars: 12g
- Fat: 10g
- Saturated Fat: 1.5g
- Sodium: 120mg

**Servings: 2**
**Cooking Time: 5 minutes**

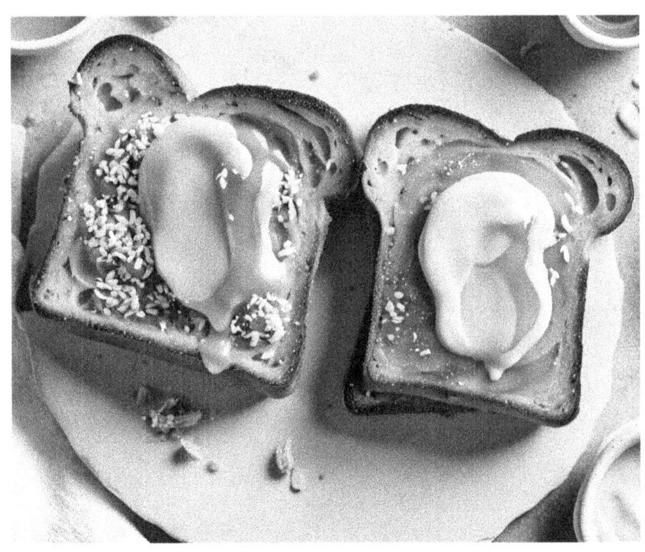

## 11. Blueberry Oat Pancakes

### Ingredients

- 1 cup rolled oats
- 1 cup unsweetened almond milk
- 1 large egg
- 1/2 cup blueberries
- 1 tablespoon honey
- 1 teaspoon baking powder
- 1/2 teaspoon ground cinnamon
- 1 teaspoon vanilla extract
- 1 tablespoon olive oil (for cooking)

### Instructions

1. In a blender, combine rolled oats, almond milk, egg, honey, baking powder, cinnamon, and vanilla extract. Blend until smooth.
2. Gently fold in the blueberries.
3. Heat a non-stick skillet over medium heat and add a small amount of olive oil.
4. Pour about 1/4 cup of the batter onto the skillet for each pancake.
5. Cook until bubbles form on the surface, then flip and cook until golden brown, about 2-3 minutes per side.
6. Repeat with the remaining batter, adding more olive oil to the skillet as needed.
7. Serve warm with additional honey or fresh blueberries if desired.

### Nutrition Info per Serving

- Calories: 280
- Protein: 8g
- Carbohydrates: 45g
- Fiber: 6g
- Sugars: 12g
- Fat: 8g
- Saturated Fat: 1g
- Sodium: 180mg

**Servings: 2**
**Cooking Time: 20 minutes**

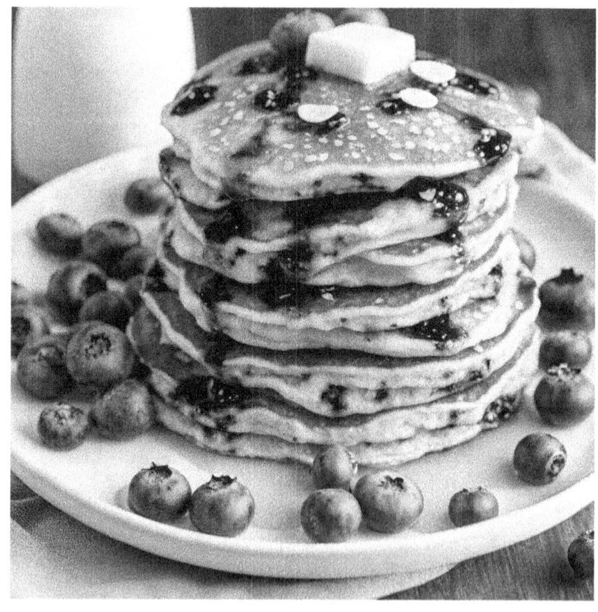

## 12. Cottage Cheese Pancakes

### Ingredients

- 1 cup cottage cheese
- 2 large eggs
- 1/2 cup rolled oats
- 1 tablespoon honey
- 1 teaspoon baking powder
- 1/2 teaspoon vanilla extract
- 1 tablespoon olive oil (for cooking)

### Instructions

1. In a blender, combine cottage cheese, eggs, oats, honey, baking powder, and vanilla extract. Blend until smooth.
2. Heat a non-stick skillet over medium heat and add a small amount of olive oil.
3. Pour about 1/4 cup of the batter onto the skillet for each pancake.
4. Cook until bubbles form on the surface, then flip and cook until golden brown, about 2-3 minutes per side.
5. Repeat with the remaining batter, adding more olive oil to the skillet as needed.
6. Serve warm with fresh fruit or a drizzle of honey if desired.

### Nutrition Info per Serving

- Calories: 250
- Protein: 18g
- Carbohydrates: 22g
- Fiber: 2g
- Sugars: 8g
- Fat: 10g
- Saturated Fat: 2g
- Sodium: 400mg

**Servings: 2**
**Cooking Time: 20 minutes**

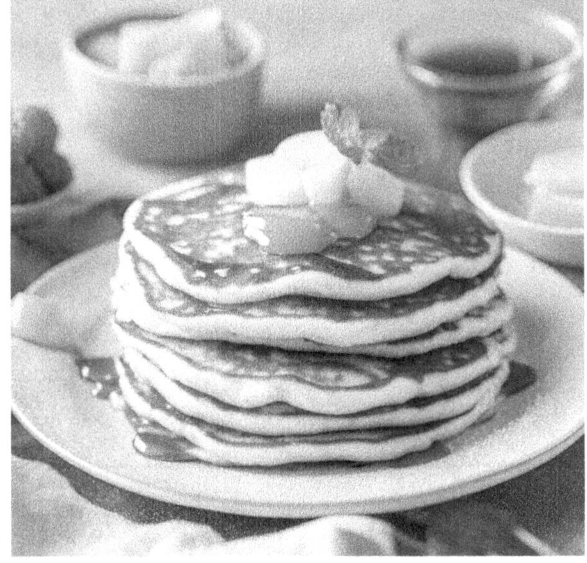

## 13. Almond Flour Waffles

### Ingredients

- 1 cup almond flour
- 2 large eggs
- 1/4 cup unsweetened almond milk
- 1 tablespoon honey
- 1 teaspoon baking powder
- 1/2 teaspoon vanilla extract
- 1 tablespoon olive oil (for cooking)

### Instructions

1. In a bowl, whisk together almond flour, eggs, almond milk, honey, baking powder, and vanilla extract until smooth.
2. Preheat a waffle iron and lightly grease with olive oil.
3. Pour the batter into the waffle iron, spreading evenly.
4. Cook according to the waffle iron instructions, usually 4-5 minutes, until golden brown.
5. Remove the waffles and serve warm with fresh fruit or a drizzle of honey if desired.

### Nutrition Info per Serving

- Calories: 300
- Protein: 12g
- Carbohydrates: 14g
- Fiber: 4g
- Sugars: 7g
- Fat: 24g
- Saturated Fat: 2g
- Sodium: 180mg

**Servings: 2**
**Cooking Time: 15 minutes**

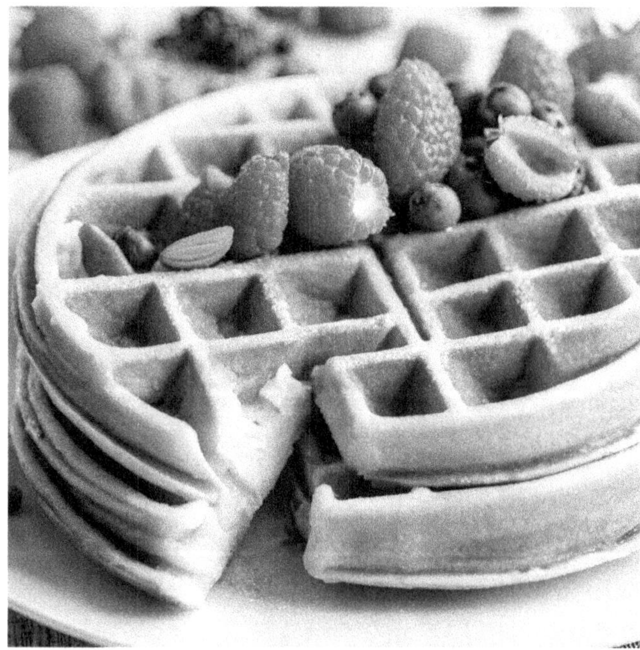

## 14. Breakfast Quinoa Bowl

**Ingredients**

- 1/2 cup quinoa, rinsed
- 1 cup water
- 1/2 cup fresh berries (strawberries, blueberries, raspberries)
- 1 small banana, sliced
- 1 tablespoon chia seeds
- 1 tablespoon honey
- 1/4 teaspoon ground cinnamon
- 1/4 cup unsweetened almond milk

**Instructions**

1. In a small pot, combine quinoa and water. Bring to a boil.
2. Reduce heat to low, cover, and simmer for about 15 minutes, or until quinoa is cooked and water is absorbed.
3. Remove from heat and let sit, covered, for 5 minutes.
4. Fluff quinoa with a fork and divide into bowls.
5. Top with fresh berries, sliced banana, chia seeds, and a drizzle of honey.
6. Sprinkle ground cinnamon on top and add a splash of almond milk.
7. Serve warm.

**Nutrition Info per Serving**

- Calories: 320
- Protein: 8g
- Carbohydrates: 62g
- Fiber: 9g
- Sugars: 20g
- Fat: 6g
- Saturated Fat: 0.5g
- Sodium: 10mg

**Servings: 2**
**Cooking Time: 20 minutes**

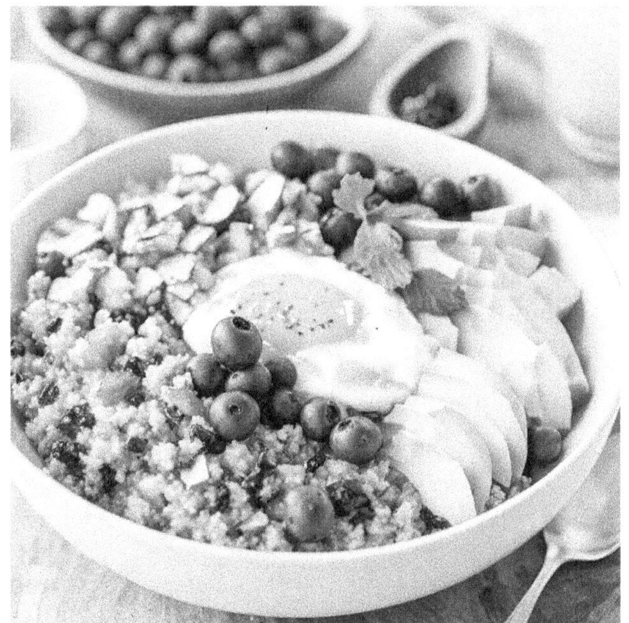

## 15. Sweet Potato Hash

**Ingredients**

- 1 large sweet potato, peeled and diced
- 1 small onion, diced
- 1 bell pepper, diced
- 1 tablespoon olive oil
- 1/2 teaspoon smoked paprika
- 1/4 teaspoon garlic powder
- 1/4 teaspoon dried thyme
- 1 tablespoon fresh parsley, chopped

**Instructions**

1. Heat olive oil in a large skillet over medium heat.
2. Add diced sweet potato, onion, and bell pepper to the skillet.
3. Cook, stirring occasionally, until the vegetables are tender and slightly crispy, about 15-20 minutes.
4. Sprinkle with smoked paprika, garlic powder, and dried thyme. Stir well to combine.
5. Cook for an additional 2-3 minutes.
6. Remove from heat and sprinkle with fresh parsley.
7. Serve warm.

**Nutrition Info per Serving**

- Calories: 200
- Protein: 3g
- Carbohydrates: 35g
- Fiber: 6g
- Sugars: 8g
- Fat: 7g
- Saturated Fat: 1g
- Sodium: 45mg

**Servings: 2**
**Cooking Time: 25 minutes**

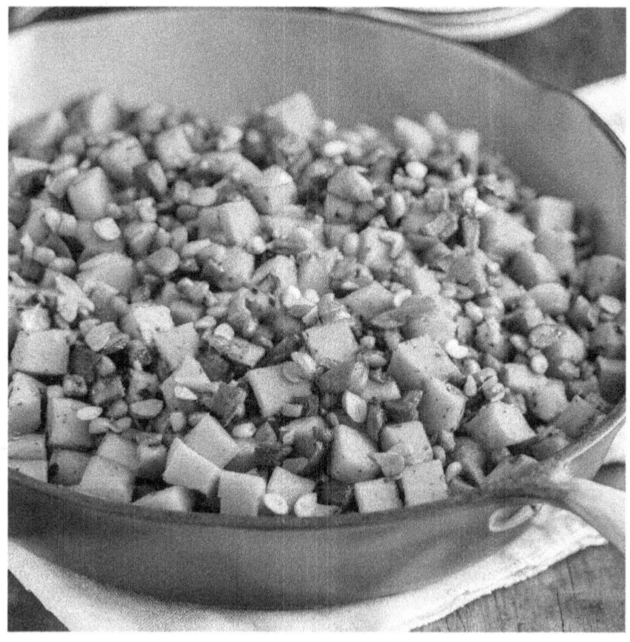

## 16. Buckwheat Porridge

**Ingredients**

- 1/2 cup buckwheat groats
- 1 cup water
- 1/2 cup unsweetened almond milk
- 1 tablespoon chia seeds
- 1 tablespoon honey
- 1/4 teaspoon ground cinnamon
- 1/4 cup chopped walnuts
- 1/4 cup fresh berries (optional)

**Instructions**

1. In a small pot, combine buckwheat groats and water. Bring to a boil.
2. Reduce heat to low, cover, and simmer for about 10-15 minutes, or until buckwheat is tender and water is absorbed.
3. Stir in almond milk, chia seeds, honey, and ground cinnamon. Cook for an additional 2-3 minutes, stirring frequently.
4. Remove from heat and let sit for a few minutes to thicken.
5. Divide porridge into bowls and top with chopped walnuts and fresh berries if desired.
6. Serve warm.

**Nutrition Info per Serving**

- Calories: 300
- Protein: 8g
- Carbohydrates: 44g
- Fiber: 8g
- Sugars: 12g
- Fat: 11g
- Saturated Fat: 1g
- Sodium: 5mg

**Servings: 2**
**Cooking Time: 20 minutes**

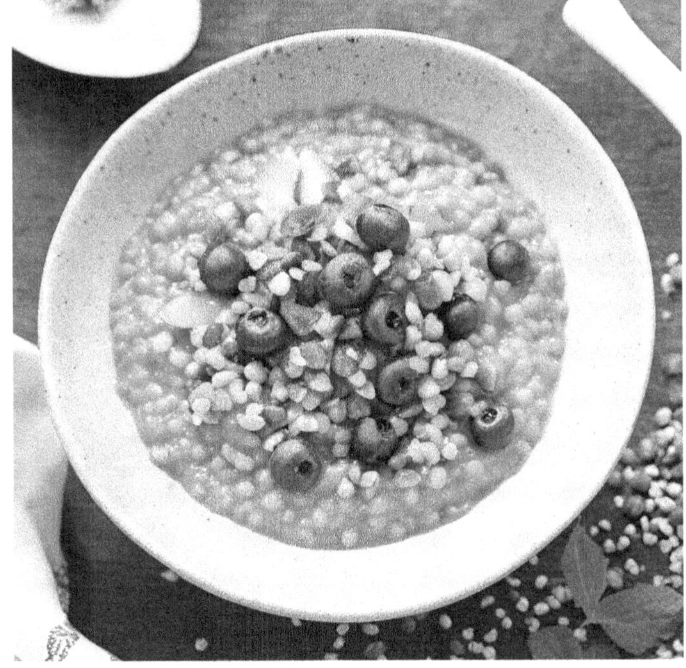

## 17. Muesli and Yogurt

**Ingredients**

- 1 cup rolled oats
- 1/4 cup chopped nuts (almonds, walnuts)
- 1/4 cup dried fruit (raisins, dried cranberries)
- 1 tablespoon chia seeds
- 1 teaspoon ground cinnamon
- 1 cup plain Greek yogurt
- 1 tablespoon honey
- 1/2 cup fresh berries (optional)

**Instructions**

1. In a large bowl, combine rolled oats, chopped nuts, dried fruit, chia seeds, and ground cinnamon. Mix well.
2. Divide the muesli mixture into bowls.
3. Top each bowl with plain Greek yogurt.
4. Drizzle honey over the yogurt.
5. Add fresh berries on top if desired.
6. Serve immediately or refrigerate for up to 24 hours.

**Nutrition Info per Serving**

- Calories: 350
- Protein: 14g
- Carbohydrates: 53g
- Fiber: 8g
- Sugars: 18g
- Fat: 11g
- Saturated Fat: 2g
- Sodium: 50mg

**Servings: 2**
**Cooking Time: 10 minutes**

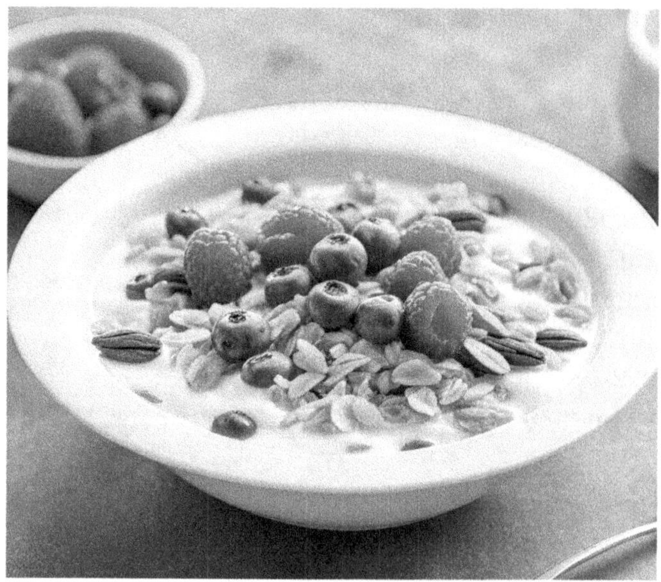

## 18. Berry and Flaxseed Yogurt

**Ingredients**

- 1 cup plain Greek yogurt
- 1/2 cup fresh mixed berries (strawberries, blueberries, raspberries)
- 1 tablespoon ground flaxseeds
- 1 tablespoon honey
- 1/4 teaspoon ground cinnamon

**Instructions**

1. In a bowl, mix the plain Greek yogurt with ground flaxseeds until well combined.
2. Top with fresh mixed berries.
3. Drizzle honey over the berries.
4. Sprinkle ground cinnamon on top.
5. Serve immediately.

**Nutrition Info per Serving**

- Calories: 250  Protein: 15g  Carbohydrates: 30g  Fiber: 6g  Sugars: 20g  Fat: 8g
- Saturated Fat: 2g  Sodium: 60mg

**Servings: 1**
**Cooking Time: 5 minutes**

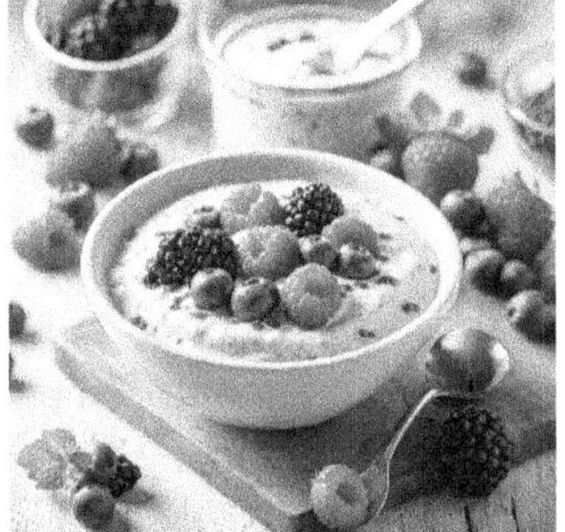

## 19. Pear and Walnut Salad

**Ingredients**

- 1 ripe pear, sliced
- 1/4 cup walnuts, chopped
- 2 cups mixed greens (spinach, arugula, kale)
- 1 tablespoon olive oil
- 1 tablespoon balsamic vinegar
- 1 teaspoon honey
- 1/4 teaspoon dried thyme

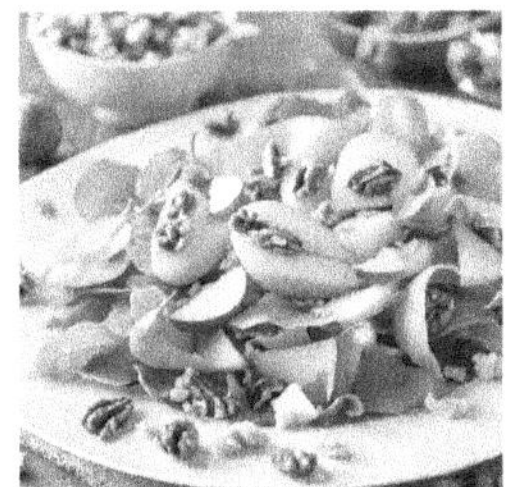

**Instructions**

1. In a small bowl, whisk together olive oil, balsamic vinegar, honey, and dried thyme to make the dressing.
2. In a large bowl, combine mixed greens, sliced pear, and chopped walnuts.
3. Drizzle the dressing over the salad and toss gently to combine.
4. Serve immediately.

**Nutrition Info per Serving**

- Calories: 230  Protein: 4g  Carbohydrates: 24g  Fiber: 5g Sugars: 14g
- Fat: 15g
- Saturated Fat: 1.5g
- Sodium: 20mg

**Servings: 2**
**Cooking Time: 10 minutes**

## 20. Peach Smoothie Bowl

**Ingredients**

- 1 cup frozen peaches
- 1 banana
- 1/2 cup unsweetened almond milk
- 1 tablespoon chia seeds
- 1 teaspoon honey
- 1/4 cup granola (no added sugar)
- 1/4 cup fresh berries (optional)

**Instructions**

1. In a blender, combine frozen peaches, banana, almond milk, chia seeds, and honey. Blend until smooth and creamy.
2. Pour the smoothie into a bowl.
3. Top with granola and fresh berries if desired.
4. Serve immediately.

**Nutrition Info per Serving**

- Calories: 280
- Protein: 5g
- Carbohydrates: 55g
- Fiber: 8g
- Sugars: 30g
- Fat: 7g
- Saturated Fat: 1g
- Sodium: 50mg

**Servings: 1**
**Cooking Time: 5 minutes**

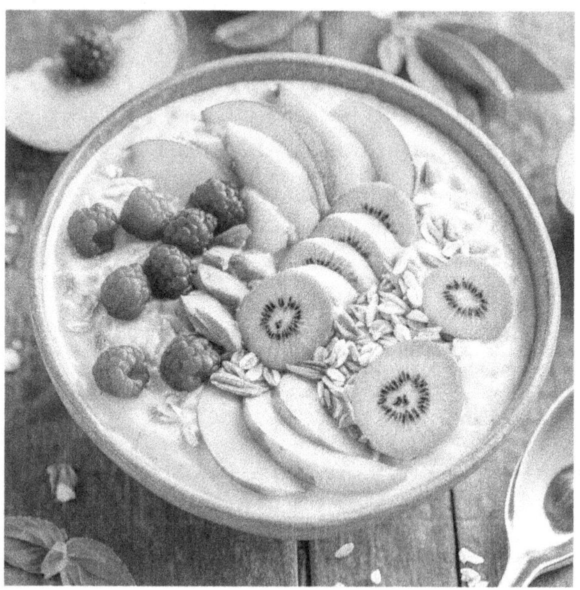

# Poultry Recipes

## 1. Grilled Chicken with Herbs

**Ingredients**

- 2 boneless, skinless chicken breasts
- 2 tablespoons olive oil
- 1 tablespoon fresh rosemary, chopped
- 1 tablespoon fresh thyme, chopped
- 1 tablespoon fresh parsley, chopped
- 1 tablespoon lemon juice
- 1 garlic clove, minced
- 1/4 teaspoon paprika

**Instructions**

1. In a small bowl, mix together olive oil, rosemary, thyme, parsley, lemon juice, minced garlic, and paprika.
2. Place the chicken breasts in a shallow dish and pour the herb mixture over them, making sure they are well coated. Marinate for at least 30 minutes in the refrigerator.
3. Preheat the grill to medium-high heat.
4. Grill the chicken breasts for 6-7 minutes on each side, or until the internal temperature reaches 165°F (75°C).
5. Remove from the grill and let rest for a few minutes before serving.

**Nutrition Info per Serving**

- Calories: 250
- Protein: 28g
- Carbohydrates: 2g
- Fiber: 0g
- Sugars: 0g
- Fat: 14g
- Saturated Fat: 2g
- Sodium: 75mg

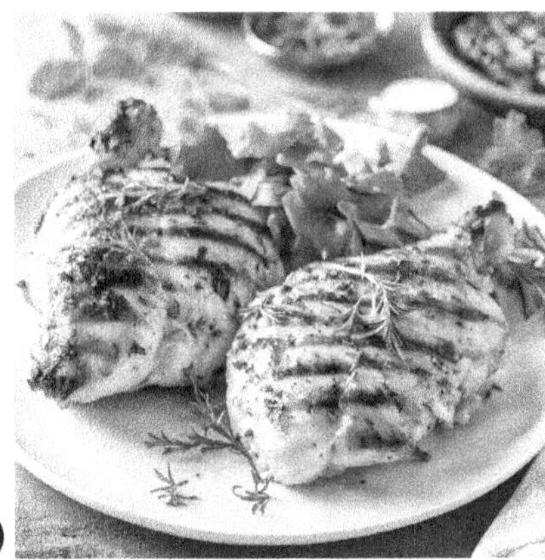

**Servings: 2**
**Cooking Time: 20 minutes (plus marinating time)**

## 2. Turkey and Spinach Meatballs

### Ingredients

- 1 pound ground turkey
- 1 cup fresh spinach, finely chopped
- 1/4 cup whole wheat breadcrumbs
- 1 egg
- 1 garlic clove, minced
- 1 tablespoon fresh parsley, chopped
- 1 teaspoon dried oregano
- 1/2 teaspoon ground cumin

### Instructions

1. Preheat the oven to 375°F (190°C) and line a baking sheet with parchment paper.
2. In a large bowl, combine ground turkey, chopped spinach, breadcrumbs, egg, minced garlic, parsley, oregano, and cumin. Mix well until all ingredients are evenly incorporated.
3. Form the mixture into 1-inch meatballs and place them on the prepared baking sheet.
4. Bake for 20-25 minutes, or until the meatballs are cooked through and golden brown.
5. Serve warm.

### Nutrition Info per Serving

- Calories: 180
- Protein: 22g
- Carbohydrates: 4g
- Fiber: 1g
- Sugars: 0g
- Fat: 9g
- Saturated Fat: 2g
- Sodium: 80mg

**Servings: 4**

**Cooking Time: 30 minutes**

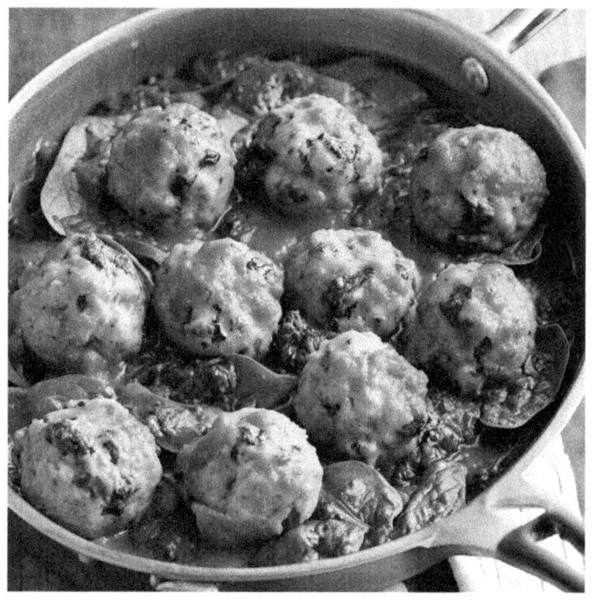

### 3. Baked Chicken with Lemon and Thyme

**Ingredients**

- 4 boneless, skinless chicken thighs
- 2 tablespoons olive oil
- 2 tablespoons lemon juice
- 1 tablespoon fresh thyme leaves
- 1 garlic clove, minced
- 1 lemon, sliced

**Instructions**

1. Preheat the oven to 375°F (190°C).
2. In a small bowl, mix together olive oil, lemon juice, thyme leaves, and minced garlic.
3. Place the chicken thighs in a baking dish and pour the olive oil mixture over them, making sure they are well coated. Arrange lemon slices on top of the chicken.
4. Bake for 30-35 minutes, or until the chicken is cooked through and the internal temperature reaches 165°F (75°C).
5. Remove from the oven and let rest for a few minutes before serving.

**Nutrition Info per Serving**

- Calories: 260
- Protein: 28g
- Carbohydrates: 2g
- Fiber: 0g
- Sugars: 0g
- Fat: 15g
- Saturated Fat: 3g
- Sodium: 85mg

**Servings: 4**
**Cooking Time: 40 minutes**

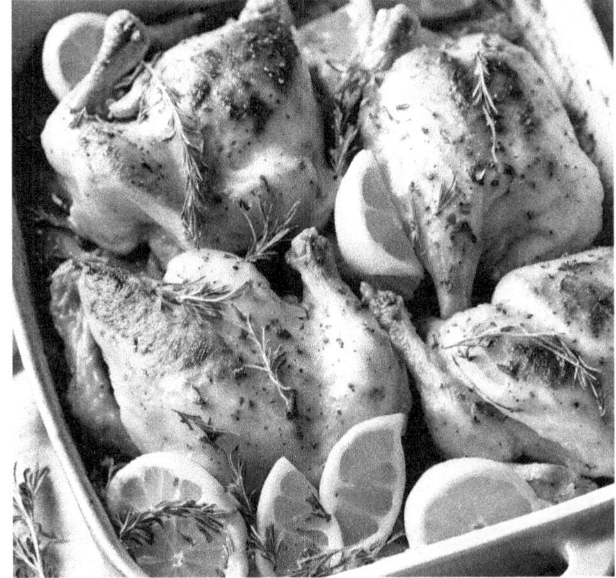

## 4. Chicken and Vegetable Soup

**Ingredients**

- 1 pound boneless, skinless chicken breasts, diced
- 1 tablespoon olive oil
- 1 onion, chopped
- 2 garlic cloves, minced
- 3 carrots, sliced
- 2 celery stalks, sliced
- 1 zucchini, diced
- 1 cup green beans, chopped
- 6 cups low-sodium chicken broth
- 1 teaspoon dried thyme
- 1 teaspoon dried basil
- 1/2 teaspoon ground turmeric

**Instructions**

1. Heat olive oil in a large pot over medium heat.
2. Add chopped onion and minced garlic. Sauté for 3-4 minutes until the onion is translucent.
3. Add diced chicken breasts and cook until the chicken is no longer pink, about 5-6 minutes.
4. Add sliced carrots, celery, zucchini, and green beans to the pot. Stir well.
5. Pour in the chicken broth and add dried thyme, basil, and turmeric.
6. Bring the soup to a boil, then reduce heat and let simmer for 20-25 minutes until the vegetables are tender.
7. Remove from heat and let sit for a few minutes before serving.

**Nutrition Info per Serving**

- Calories: 220
- Protein: 25g
- Carbohydrates: 15g
- Fiber: 4g
- Sugars: 6g
- Fat: 7g
- Saturated Fat: 1.5g
- Sodium: 200mg

**Servings: 6**
**Cooking Time: 45 minutes**

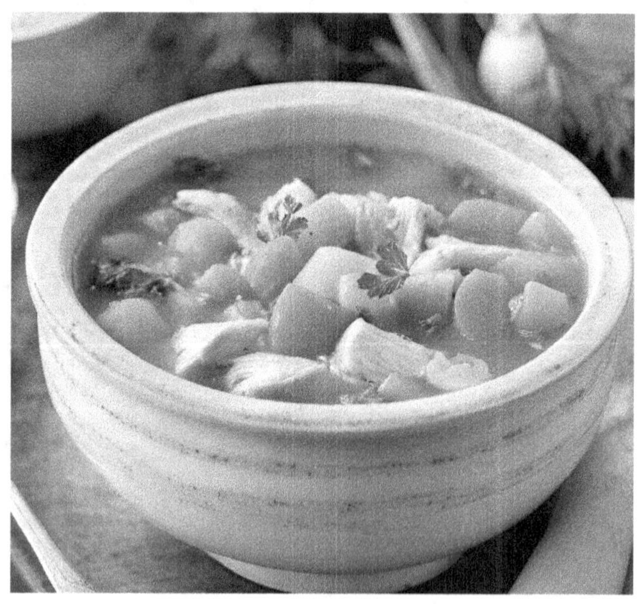

## 5. Oven-Roasted Turkey Breast

### Ingredients

- 1 boneless turkey breast (about 2 pounds)
- 2 tablespoons olive oil
- 1 tablespoon fresh rosemary, chopped
- 1 tablespoon fresh thyme, chopped
- 2 garlic cloves, minced
- 1 lemon, zested and juiced
- 1/4 teaspoon paprika

### Instructions

1. Preheat the oven to 375°F (190°C).
2. In a small bowl, mix together olive oil, rosemary, thyme, garlic, lemon zest, lemon juice, and paprika.
3. Rub the mixture all over the turkey breast.
4. Place the turkey breast on a roasting pan and roast in the preheated oven for 45-60 minutes, or until the internal temperature reaches 165°F (75°C).
5. Remove from the oven and let rest for 10 minutes before slicing.
6. Serve warm.

### Nutrition Info per Serving

- Calories: 250
- Protein: 28g
- Carbohydrates: 2g
- Fiber: 0g
- Sugars: 0g
- Fat: 14g
- Saturated Fat: 2g
- Sodium: 70mg

**Servings: 4**
**Cooking Time: 60 minutes**

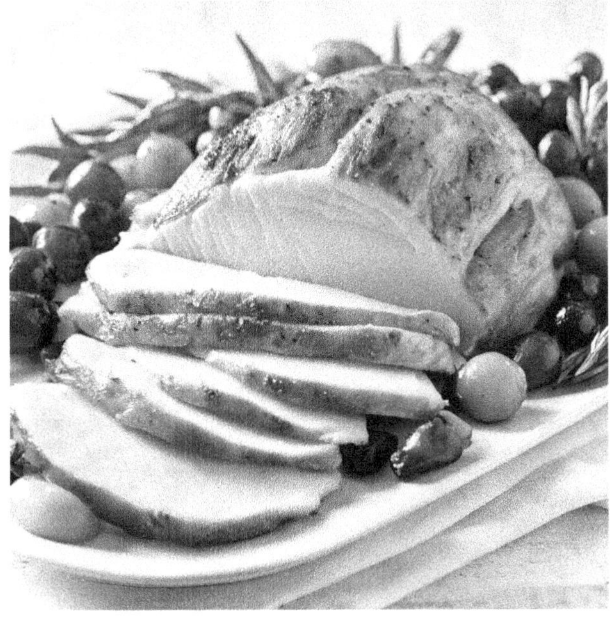

## 6. Chicken Salad with Avocado

### Ingredients

- 2 boneless, skinless chicken breasts, cooked and shredded
- 1 ripe avocado, diced
- 1/2 cup cherry tomatoes, halved
- 1/4 cup red onion, finely chopped
- 2 tablespoons fresh cilantro, chopped
- 1 tablespoon lime juice
- 1 tablespoon olive oil
- 1/4 teaspoon ground cumin

### Instructions

1. In a large bowl, combine shredded chicken, diced avocado, cherry tomatoes, red onion, and cilantro.
2. In a small bowl, whisk together lime juice, olive oil, and ground cumin.
3. Pour the dressing over the salad and toss gently to combine.
4. Serve immediately.

### Nutrition Info per Serving

- Calories: 290
- Protein: 25g
- Carbohydrates: 10g
- Fiber: 6g
- Sugars: 2g
- Fat: 18g
- Saturated Fat: 3g
- Sodium: 50mg

### Servings: 2
### Cooking Time: 20 minutes

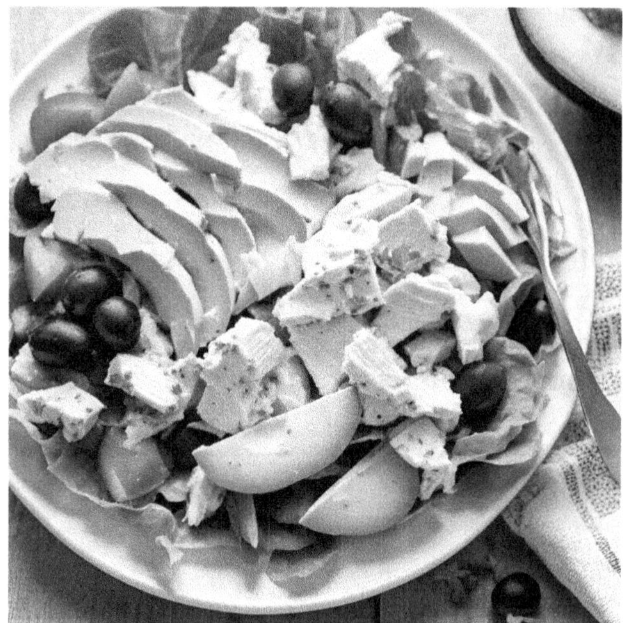

## 7. Ground Turkey Stuffed Peppers

### Ingredients

- 4 large bell peppers, tops cut off and seeds removed
- 1 pound ground turkey
- 1 cup cooked quinoa
- 1 small onion, diced
- 2 garlic cloves, minced
- 1 cup diced tomatoes
- 1 teaspoon dried oregano
- 1 teaspoon ground cumin
- 1 tablespoon olive oil

### Instructions

1. Preheat the oven to 375°F (190°C).
2. Heat olive oil in a large skillet over medium heat.
3. Add diced onion and minced garlic to the skillet. Cook until the onion is translucent, about 3-4 minutes.
4. Add ground turkey to the skillet and cook until no longer pink, about 5-6 minutes.
5. Stir in cooked quinoa, diced tomatoes, oregano, and cumin. Cook for an additional 2-3 minutes.
6. Stuff the bell peppers with the turkey mixture and place them in a baking dish.
7. Cover with foil and bake for 30 minutes.
8. Remove the foil and bake for an additional 10 minutes, until the peppers are tender.
9. Serve warm.

### Nutrition Info per Serving

- Calories: 280
- Protein: 26g
- Carbohydrates: 20g
- Fiber: 5g
- Sugars: 7g
- Fat: 11g
- Saturated Fat: 2g
- Sodium: 80mg

**Servings: 4**
**Cooking Time: 45 minutes**

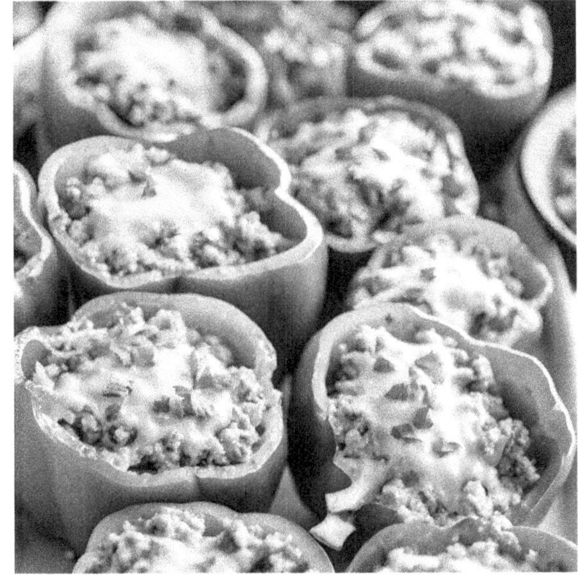

## 8. Chicken and Broccoli Stir-fry

**Ingredients**

- 2 boneless, skinless chicken breasts, sliced thinly
- 2 cups broccoli florets
- 1 red bell pepper, sliced
- 1 small onion, sliced
- 2 garlic cloves, minced
- 1 tablespoon olive oil
- 1 tablespoon low-sodium soy sauce
- 1 teaspoon ground ginger
- 1/2 teaspoon garlic powder

**Instructions**

1. Heat olive oil in a large skillet or wok over medium-high heat.
2. Add sliced chicken to the skillet and cook until no longer pink, about 5-6 minutes.
3. Add minced garlic, broccoli, bell pepper, and onion to the skillet. Stir-fry for about 4-5 minutes, until the vegetables are tender.
4. Stir in soy sauce, ground ginger, and garlic powder. Cook for an additional 2 minutes.
5. Remove from heat and serve immediately.

**Nutrition Info per Serving**

- Calories: 220
- Protein: 25g
- Carbohydrates: 12g
- Fiber: 4g
- Sugars: 5g
- Fat: 8g
- Saturated Fat: 1.5g
- Sodium: 200mg

**Servings: 2**
**Cooking Time: 20 minutes**

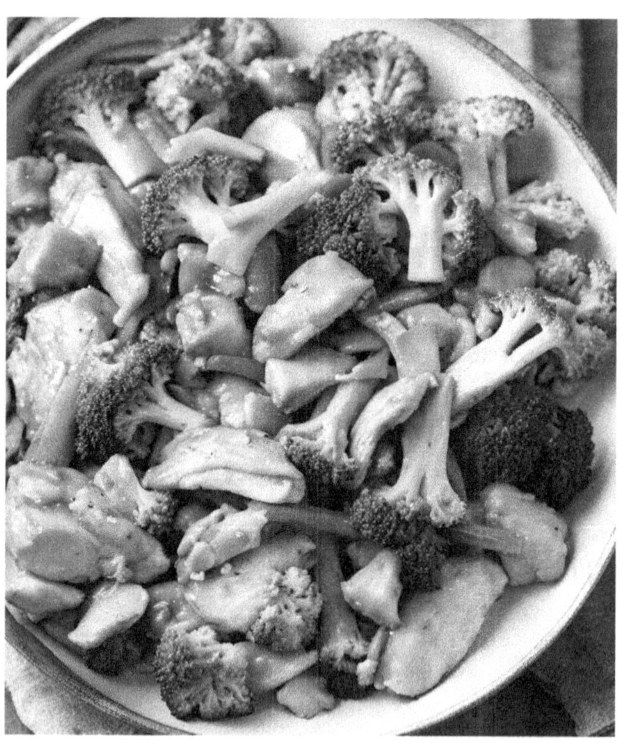

## 9. Poached Chicken and Quinoa Salad

### Ingredients

- 2 boneless, skinless chicken breasts
- 1 cup quinoa
- 2 cups water or low-sodium chicken broth
- 1/2 cup cherry tomatoes, halved
- 1/2 cucumber, diced
- 1/4 cup red onion, finely chopped
- 2 tablespoons fresh parsley, chopped
- 1 tablespoon lemon juice
- 1 tablespoon olive oil
- 1/4 teaspoon ground cumin

### Instructions

1. In a medium pot, bring water or chicken broth to a boil.
2. Add chicken breasts and reduce heat to a simmer. Poach the chicken for about 15-20 minutes, or until cooked through.
3. Remove the chicken from the pot and let cool slightly before shredding.
4. In another pot, cook quinoa according to package instructions, using water or chicken broth.
5. In a large bowl, combine cooked quinoa, shredded chicken, cherry tomatoes, cucumber, red onion, and parsley.
6. In a small bowl, whisk together lemon juice, olive oil, and ground cumin.
7. Pour the dressing over the salad and toss gently to combine.
8. Serve immediately.

### Nutrition Info per Serving

- Calories: 290
- Protein: 28g
- Carbohydrates: 24g
- Fiber: 4g
- Sugars: 4g
- Fat: 10g
- Saturated Fat: 1.5g
- Sodium: 75mg

**Servings: 2**
**Cooking Time: 35 minutes**

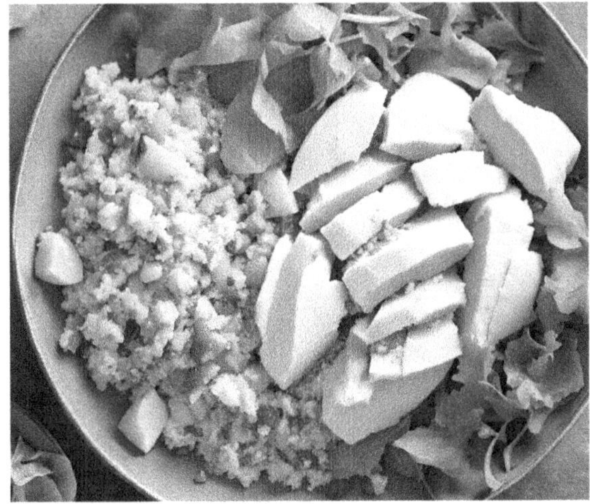

## 10. Spicy Grilled Turkey Burgers

**Ingredients**

- 1 pound ground turkey
- 1/4 cup finely chopped onion
- 1 garlic clove, minced
- 1 teaspoon ground cumin
- 1/2 teaspoon ground paprika
- 1/4 teaspoon cayenne pepper
- 1 tablespoon fresh parsley, chopped
- 1 tablespoon olive oil

**Instructions**

1. In a large bowl, combine ground turkey, chopped onion, minced garlic, cumin, paprika, cayenne pepper, and parsley. Mix well until all ingredients are evenly incorporated.
2. Form the mixture into 4 equal patties.
3. Preheat the grill to medium-high heat and lightly brush with olive oil.
4. Grill the turkey burgers for 5-6 minutes on each side, or until the internal temperature reaches 165°F (75°C).
5. Remove from the grill and let rest for a few minutes before serving.

**Nutrition Info per Serving**

- Calories: 210
- Protein: 22g
- Carbohydrates: 2g
- Fiber: 0.5g
- Sugars: 0g
- Fat: 12g
- Saturated Fat: 2g
- Sodium: 60mg

**Servings: 4**
**Cooking Time: 20 minutes**

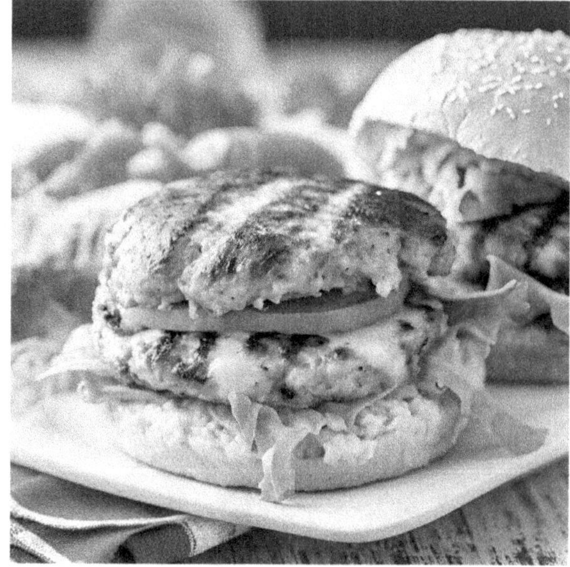

## 11. Chicken Tikka Skewers

### Ingredients

- 1 pound boneless, skinless chicken breasts, cut into cubes
- 1/2 cup plain Greek yogurt
- 1 tablespoon lemon juice
- 1 tablespoon fresh ginger, minced
- 2 garlic cloves, minced
- 1 teaspoon ground cumin
- 1 teaspoon ground coriander
- 1/2 teaspoon ground turmeric
- 1/2 teaspoon ground paprika
- 1/4 teaspoon cayenne pepper
- 1 tablespoon olive oil

### Instructions

1. In a large bowl, mix together Greek yogurt, lemon juice, minced ginger, minced garlic, cumin, coriander, turmeric, paprika, and cayenne pepper.
2. Add the chicken cubes to the bowl and toss to coat evenly. Marinate for at least 30 minutes in the refrigerator.
3. Preheat the grill to medium-high heat and lightly brush with olive oil.
4. Thread the marinated chicken cubes onto skewers.
5. Grill the skewers for 5-7 minutes on each side, or until the chicken is cooked through and has a slight char.
6. Remove from the grill and serve immediately.

### Nutrition Info per Serving

- Calories: 200
- Protein: 28g
- Carbohydrates: 4g
- Fiber: 0.5g
- Sugars: 2g
- Fat: 8g
- Saturated Fat: 2g
- Sodium: 70mg

**Servings: 4**
**Cooking Time: 25 minutes**
**(plus marinating time)**

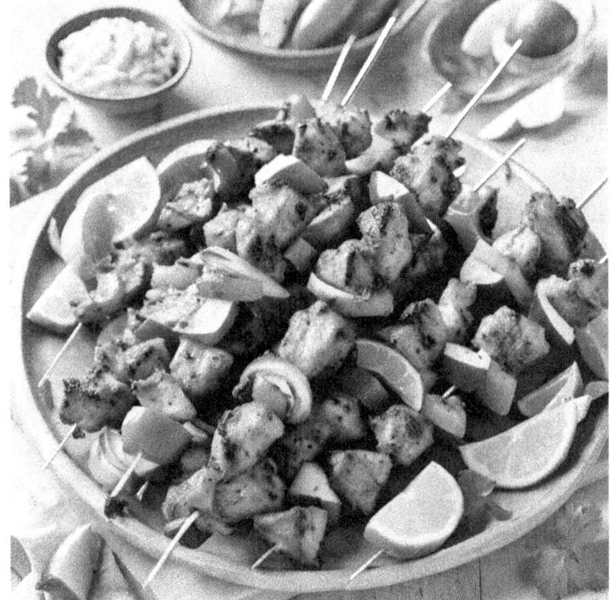

## 12. Ground Chicken and Vegetable Skillet

### Ingredients

- 1 pound ground chicken
- 1 zucchini, diced
- 1 bell pepper, diced
- 1 small onion, diced
- 2 garlic cloves, minced
- 1 cup cherry tomatoes, halved
- 1 teaspoon dried oregano
- 1/2 teaspoon ground cumin
- 1 tablespoon olive oil

### Instructions

1. Heat olive oil in a large skillet over medium heat.
2. Add diced onion and minced garlic. Sauté for 2-3 minutes until the onion is translucent.
3. Add ground chicken to the skillet and cook until no longer pink, about 5-6 minutes.
4. Add diced zucchini, bell pepper, and cherry tomatoes to the skillet. Cook for an additional 5-6 minutes, until the vegetables are tender.
5. Stir in dried oregano and ground cumin. Cook for another 2-3 minutes.
6. Remove from heat and serve immediately.

### Nutrition Info per Serving

- Calories: 220
- Protein: 25g
- Carbohydrates: 10g
- Fiber: 3g
- Sugars: 5g
- Fat: 10g
- Saturated Fat: 2g
- Sodium: 75mg

**Servings: 4**
**Cooking Time: 25 minutes**

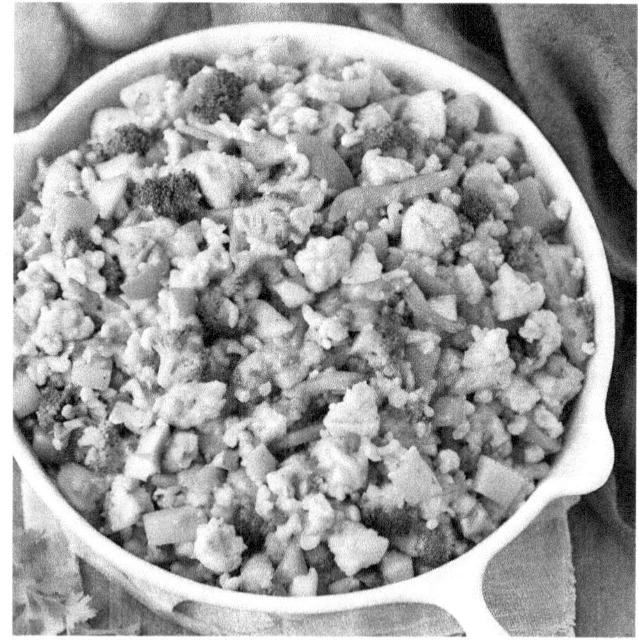

**13. Turkey and Sweet Potato Hash**

**Ingredients**

- 1 pound ground turkey
- 2 medium sweet potatoes, peeled and diced
- 1 small onion, diced
- 1 bell pepper, diced
- 2 garlic cloves, minced
- 1 teaspoon ground cumin
- 1/2 teaspoon smoked paprika
- 1 tablespoon olive oil
- 1 tablespoon fresh parsley, chopped

**Instructions**

1. Heat olive oil in a large skillet over medium heat.
2. Add diced sweet potatoes to the skillet and cook for about 10 minutes, stirring occasionally, until they begin to soften.
3. Add diced onion, bell pepper, and minced garlic. Cook for an additional 5 minutes.
4. Push the vegetables to one side of the skillet and add ground turkey. Cook until no longer pink, about 5-6 minutes.
5. Stir in ground cumin and smoked paprika. Mix well to combine.
6. Cook for another 2-3 minutes until everything is heated through and well mixed.
7. Remove from heat and sprinkle with fresh parsley.
8. Serve warm.

**Nutrition Info per Serving**

- Calories: 280
- Protein: 26g
- Carbohydrates: 22g
- Fiber: 5g
- Sugars: 6g
- Fat: 11g
- Saturated Fat: 2g
- Sodium: 80mg

**Servings: 4**
**Cooking Time: 30 minutes**

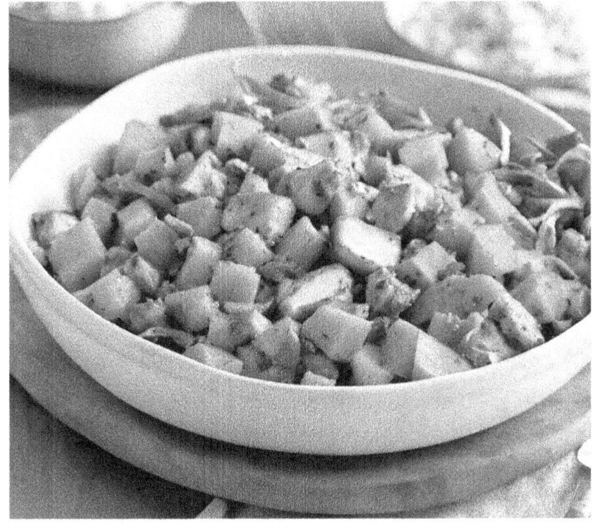

## 14. Baked Chicken with Ratatouille

**Ingredients**

- 4 boneless, skinless chicken breasts
- 1 zucchini, diced
- 1 eggplant, diced
- 1 bell pepper, diced
- 1 onion, diced
- 2 garlic cloves, minced
- 1 can (14.5 oz) diced tomatoes
- 1 teaspoon dried basil
- 1 teaspoon dried oregano
- 1 tablespoon olive oil

**Instructions**

1. Preheat the oven to 375°F (190°C).
2. Heat olive oil in a large skillet over medium heat.
3. Add diced onion and minced garlic. Sauté for 2-3 minutes until the onion is translucent.
4. Add diced zucchini, eggplant, bell pepper, and canned tomatoes (with juice) to the skillet. Stir in dried basil and oregano.
5. Cook for about 10 minutes, until the vegetables are tender.
6. Place the chicken breasts in a baking dish and pour the vegetable mixture over them.
7. Cover the baking dish with foil and bake for 25-30 minutes, or until the chicken is cooked through and the internal temperature reaches 165°F (75°C).
8. Remove from the oven and let rest for a few minutes before serving.

**Nutrition Info per Serving**

- Calories: 300
- Protein: 30g
- Carbohydrates: 15g
- Fiber: 6g
- Sugars: 8g
- Fat: 12g
- Saturated Fat: 2g
- Sodium: 200mg

**Servings: 4**
**Cooking Time: 40 minutes**

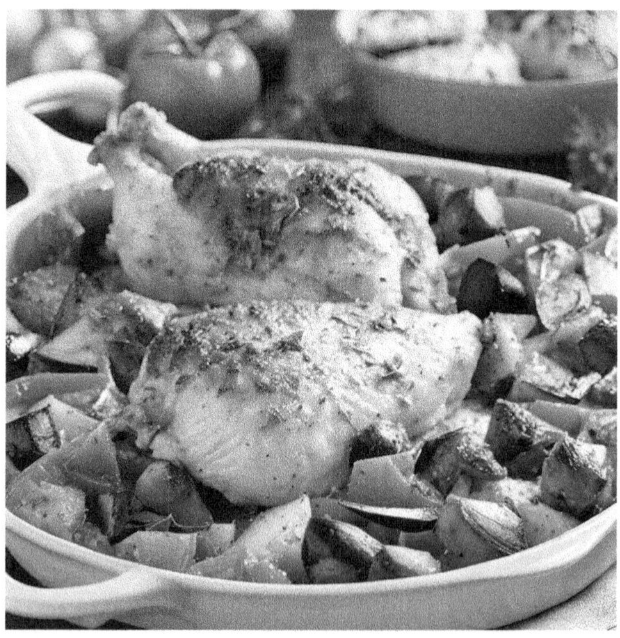

**15. Turkey Meatloaf with Mushrooms**
**Ingredients**

- 1 pound ground turkey
- 1 cup mushrooms, finely chopped
- 1 small onion, finely chopped
- 1 garlic clove, minced
- 1/2 cup whole wheat breadcrumbs
- 1 egg
- 1 tablespoon fresh parsley, chopped
- 1 teaspoon dried thyme
- 1 tablespoon olive oil

**Instructions**

1. Preheat the oven to 375°F (190°C).
2. In a skillet, heat olive oil over medium heat. Add chopped onions and minced garlic, and sauté until translucent, about 3-4 minutes.
3. Add chopped mushrooms to the skillet and cook until they release their moisture and become tender, about 5-6 minutes. Remove from heat and let cool slightly.
4. In a large bowl, combine ground turkey, cooked mushroom mixture, breadcrumbs, egg, parsley, and thyme. Mix until well combined.
5. Transfer the mixture to a loaf pan and shape into a loaf.
6. Bake in the preheated oven for 45-50 minutes, or until the internal temperature reaches 165°F (75°C).
7. Remove from the oven and let rest for 10 minutes before slicing.
8. Serve warm.

**Nutrition Info per Serving**

- Calories: 220
- Protein: 25g
- Carbohydrates: 10g
- Fiber: 2g
- Sugars: 3g
- Fat: 9g
- Saturated Fat: 2g
- Sodium: 80mg

**Servings: 4**
**Cooking Time: 60 minutes**

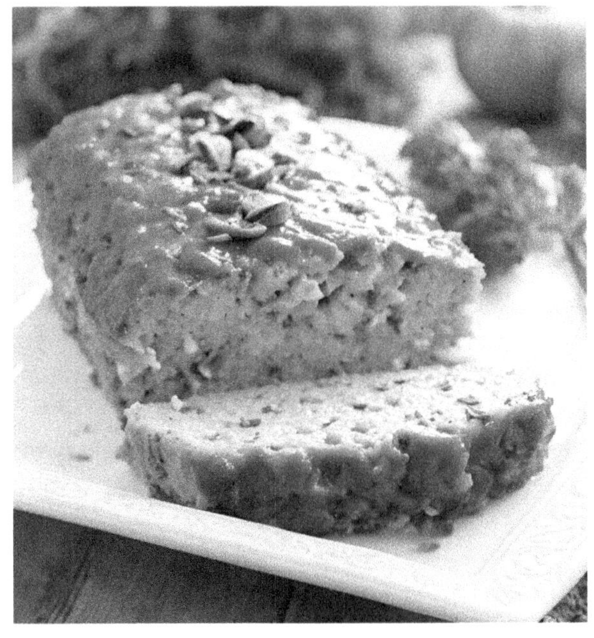

## 16. Chicken Cacciatore

**Ingredients**

- 4 boneless, skinless chicken thighs
- 1 tablespoon olive oil
- 1 small onion, diced
- 2 garlic cloves, minced
- 1 bell pepper, sliced
- 1 can (14.5 oz) diced tomatoes
- 1 cup sliced mushrooms
- 1/2 cup chicken broth
- 1 teaspoon dried oregano
- 1 teaspoon dried basil
- 1/4 teaspoon ground black pepper

**Instructions**

1. Heat olive oil in a large skillet over medium heat.
2. Add chicken thighs and cook until browned on both sides, about 5 minutes per side. Remove chicken from the skillet and set aside.
3. In the same skillet, add diced onion and minced garlic. Sauté until the onion is translucent, about 3-4 minutes.
4. Add bell pepper and mushrooms to the skillet and cook until tender, about 5-6 minutes.
5. Stir in diced tomatoes, chicken broth, oregano, basil, and ground black pepper.
6. Return the chicken thighs to the skillet and bring to a simmer.
7. Cover and cook for 30-35 minutes, until the chicken is cooked through and tender.
8. Remove from heat and serve warm.

**Nutrition Info per Serving**

- Calories: 250
- Protein: 26g
- Carbohydrates: 12g
- Fiber: 3g
- Sugars: 7g
- Fat: 12g
- Saturated Fat: 2g
- Sodium: 200mg

**Servings: 4**

**Cooking Time: 45 minutes**

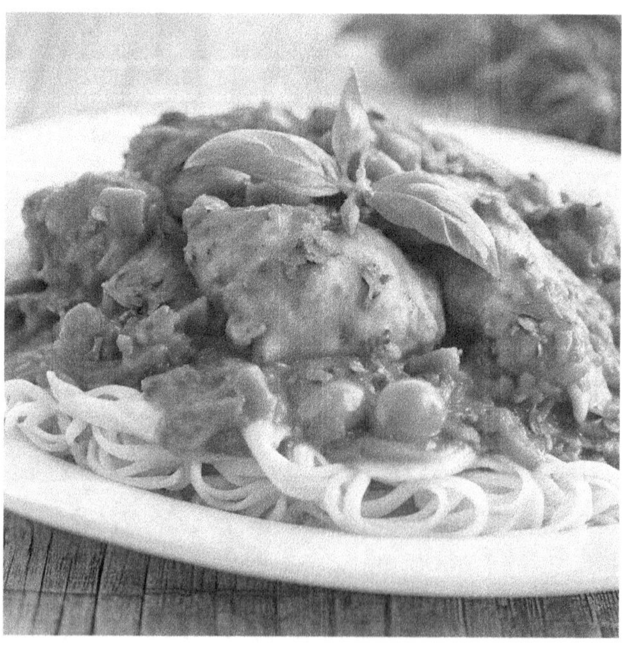

**17. Turkey and Zucchini Burgers**

**Ingredients**

- 1 pound ground turkey
- 1 cup grated zucchini
- 1 small onion, finely chopped
- 1 garlic clove, minced
- 1 egg
- 1/4 cup whole wheat breadcrumbs
- 1 teaspoon dried oregano
- 1 tablespoon olive oil

Instructions

1. In a large bowl, combine ground turkey, grated zucchini, chopped onion, minced garlic, egg, breadcrumbs, and oregano. Mix until well combined.
2. Form the mixture into 4 equal patties.
3. Heat olive oil in a non-stick skillet over medium heat.
4. Cook the patties for about 5-6 minutes on each side, or until the internal temperature reaches 165°F (75°C).
5. Remove from the skillet and let rest for a few minutes before serving.

**Nutrition Info per Serving**

- Calories: 230
- Protein: 25g
- Carbohydrates: 10g
- Fiber: 2g
- Sugars: 3g
- Fat: 10g
- Saturated Fat: 2g
- Sodium: 75mg

**Servings: 4**
**Cooking Time: 20 minutes**

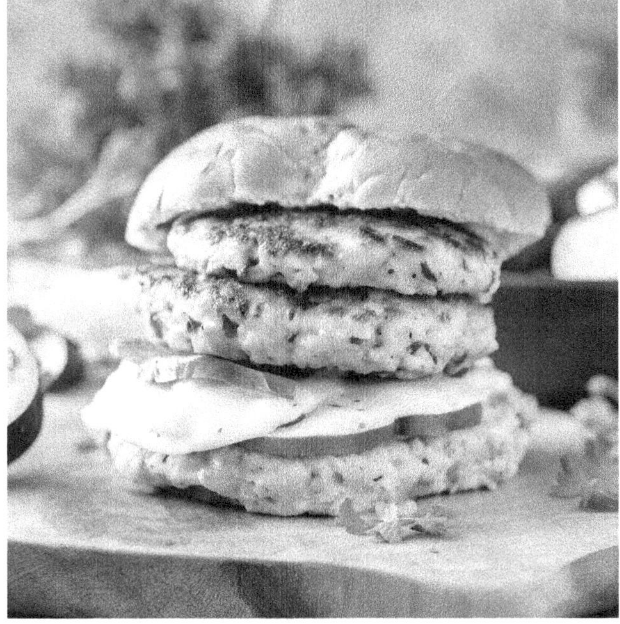

## 18. Baked Tandoori Chicken

**Ingredients**

- 4 boneless, skinless chicken breasts
- 1 cup plain Greek yogurt
- 1 tablespoon lemon juice
- 1 tablespoon fresh ginger, minced
- 2 garlic cloves, minced
- 1 teaspoon ground cumin
- 1 teaspoon ground coriander
- 1/2 teaspoon ground turmeric
- 1/2 teaspoon ground paprika
- 1/4 teaspoon cayenne pepper
- 1 tablespoon olive oil

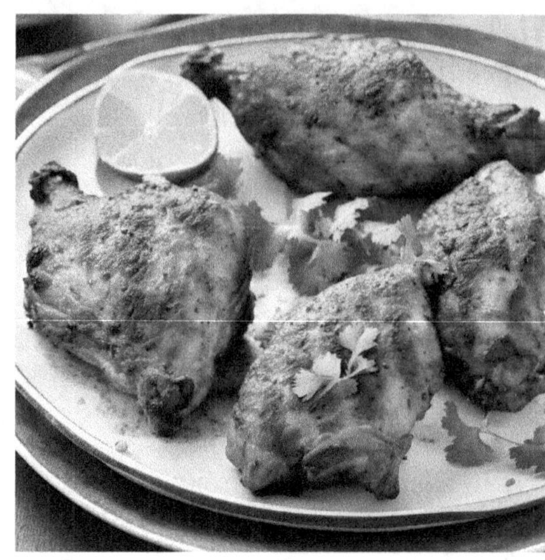

**Instructions**

1. In a large bowl, mix together Greek yogurt, lemon juice, minced ginger, minced garlic, cumin, coriander, turmeric, paprika, and cayenne pepper.
2. Add the chicken breasts to the bowl and toss to coat evenly. Marinate for at least 1 hour in the refrigerator.
3. Preheat the oven to 375°F (190°C).
4. Place the marinated chicken breasts on a baking sheet lined with parchment paper.
5. Bake in the preheated oven for 25-30 minutes, or until the internal temperature reaches 165°F (75°C).
6. Remove from the oven and let rest for a few minutes before serving.

**Nutrition Info per Serving**

- Calories: 260
- Protein: 28g
- Carbohydrates: 8g
- Fiber: 1g
- Sugars: 4g
- Fat: 12g
- Saturated Fat: 2g
- Sodium: 100mg

**Servings: 4**

**Cooking Time: 40 minutes (plus marinating time)**

**19. Creamy Chicken and Mushroom Soup**

**Ingredients**

- 1 pound boneless, skinless chicken breasts, diced
- 2 tablespoons olive oil
- 1 small onion, diced
- 2 garlic cloves, minced
- 2 cups sliced mushrooms
- 4 cups low-sodium chicken broth
- 1 cup unsweetened almond milk
- 1 teaspoon dried thyme
- 1/2 teaspoon ground black pepper
- 2 tablespoons whole wheat flour
- 1 tablespoon fresh parsley, chopped

**Instructions**

1. Heat olive oil in a large pot over medium heat.
2. Add diced onion and minced garlic. Sauté until the onion is translucent, about 3-4 minutes.
3. Add diced chicken and cook until no longer pink, about 5-6 minutes.
4. Add sliced mushrooms and cook for an additional 3-4 minutes until tender.
5. Stir in whole wheat flour and cook for 1-2 minutes to form a roux.
6. Gradually add chicken broth while stirring to avoid lumps. Bring to a boil.
7. Reduce heat to a simmer and add thyme and ground black pepper.
8. Stir in almond milk and let the soup simmer for 15-20 minutes until thickened.
9. Remove from heat and stir in fresh parsley.
10. Serve warm.

**Nutrition Info per Serving**

- Calories: 250
- Protein: 25g
- Carbohydrates: 10g
- Fiber: 2g
- Sugars: 3g
- Fat: 12g
- Saturated Fat: 2g
- Sodium: 150mg

**Servings: 4**

**Cooking Time: 35 minutes**

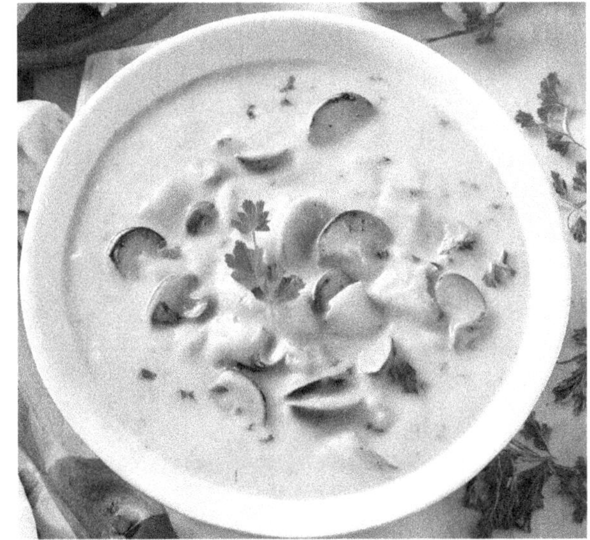

## 20. Turkey and Kale Soup

### Ingredients

- 1 pound ground turkey
- 1 tablespoon olive oil
- 1 small onion, diced
- 2 garlic cloves, minced
- 2 carrots, sliced
- 2 celery stalks, sliced
- 4 cups low-sodium chicken broth
- 2 cups chopped kale
- 1 teaspoon dried thyme
- 1/2 teaspoon ground cumin

### Instructions

1. Heat olive oil in a large pot over medium heat.
2. Add diced onion and minced garlic. Sauté until the onion is translucent, about 3-4 minutes.
3. Add ground turkey and cook until no longer pink, about 5-6 minutes.
4. Add sliced carrots and celery to the pot and cook for an additional 5 minutes.
5. Pour in chicken broth and bring to a boil.
6. Reduce heat to a simmer and add chopped kale, thyme, and cumin.
7. Let the soup simmer for 20-25 minutes until vegetables are tender.
8. Remove from heat and serve warm.

### Nutrition Info per Serving

- Calories: 220
- Protein: 22g
- Carbohydrates: 10g
- Fiber: 3g
- Sugars: 4g
- Fat: 10g
- Saturated Fat: 2g
- Sodium: 150mg

**Servings: 4**
**Cooking Time: 35 minutes**

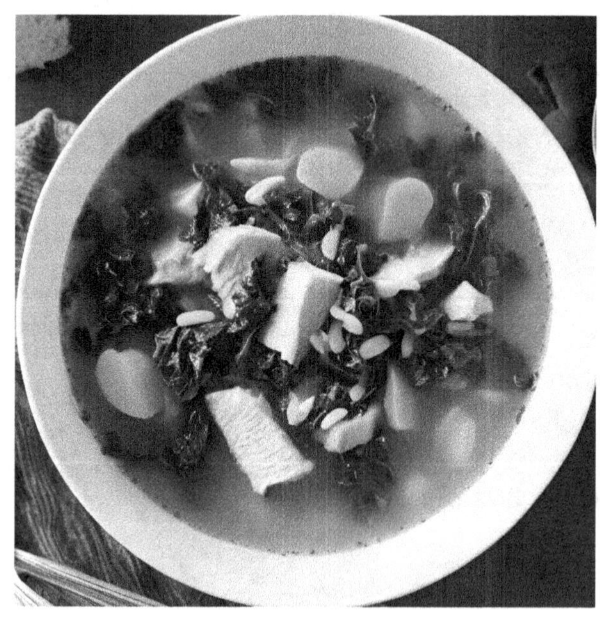

# 21. Sautéed Chicken with Spinach and Pine Nuts

## Ingredients

- 2 boneless, skinless chicken breasts, sliced thinly
- 1 tablespoon olive oil
- 2 garlic cloves, minced
- 4 cups fresh spinach
- 2 tablespoons pine nuts
- 1 tablespoon lemon juice
- 1/4 teaspoon ground black pepper

## Instructions

1. Heat olive oil in a large skillet over medium heat.
2. Add sliced chicken to the skillet and cook until no longer pink, about 5-6 minutes.
3. Add minced garlic and cook for an additional 1-2 minutes.
4. Add fresh spinach to the skillet and cook until wilted, about 2-3 minutes.
5. Stir in pine nuts, lemon juice, and ground black pepper.
6. Cook for an additional 1-2 minutes until everything is heated through.
7. Remove from heat and serve warm.

## Nutrition Info per Serving

- Calories: 220
- Protein: 26g
- Carbohydrates: 4g
- Fiber: 2g
- Sugars: 1g
- Fat: 12g
- Saturated Fat: 2g
- Sodium: 75mg

**Servings: 2**
**Cooking Time: 20 minutes**

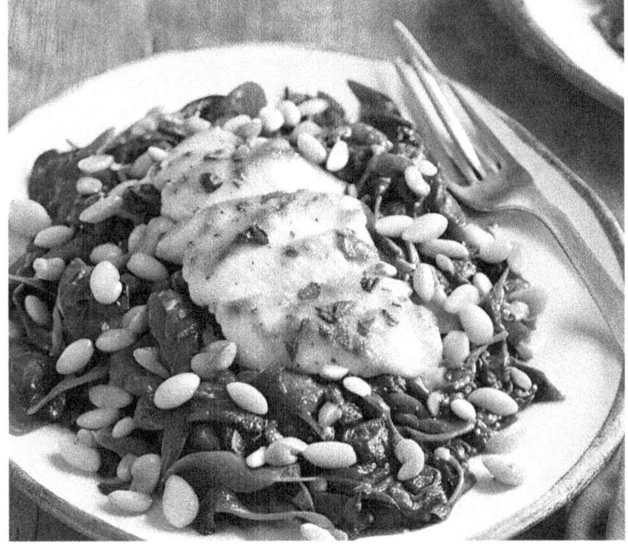

## 22. Stuffed Chicken Breast with Spinach and Ricotta

### Ingredients

- 2 boneless, skinless chicken breasts
- 1/2 cup ricotta cheese
- 1 cup fresh spinach, chopped
- 1 garlic clove, minced
- 1 tablespoon olive oil
- 1/4 teaspoon ground black pepper
- 1 tablespoon fresh basil, chopped

### Instructions

1. Preheat the oven to 375°F (190°C).
2. In a bowl, mix together ricotta cheese, chopped spinach, minced garlic, ground black pepper, and chopped basil.
3. Cut a pocket into each chicken breast and stuff with the ricotta mixture.
4. Secure with toothpicks if necessary.
5. Heat olive oil in a skillet over medium heat and sear the chicken breasts for 2-3 minutes on each side until golden brown.
6. Transfer the chicken to a baking dish and bake in the preheated oven for 20-25 minutes, or until the internal temperature reaches 165°F (75°C).
7. Remove from the oven and let rest for a few minutes before serving.

### Nutrition Info per Serving

- Calories: 280
- Protein: 32g
- Carbohydrates: 4g
- Fiber: 1g
- Sugars: 1g
- Fat: 14g
- Saturated Fat: 5g
- Sodium: 150mg

**Servings: 2**
**Cooking Time: 30 minutes**

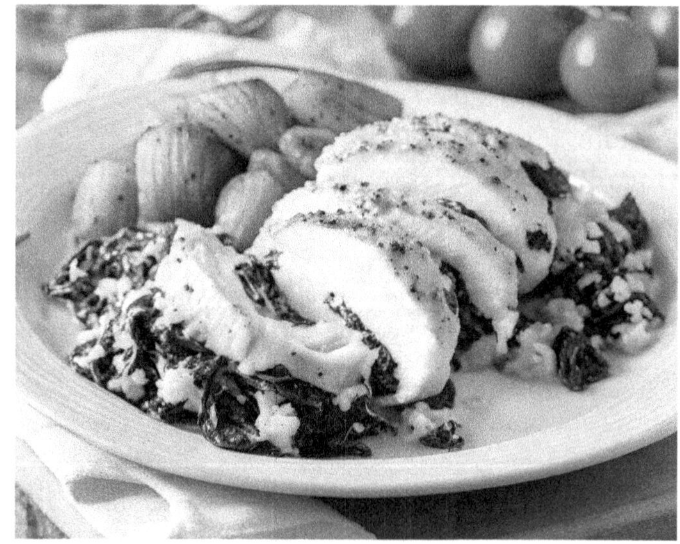

## 23. Ground Turkey and Cauliflower Rice Bowl

**Ingredients**

- 1 pound ground turkey
- 1 tablespoon olive oil
- 1 small onion, diced
- 2 garlic cloves, minced
- 1 bell pepper, diced
- 1 cup cauliflower rice
- 1 teaspoon ground cumin
- 1/2 teaspoon ground turmeric
- 1/4 teaspoon ground black pepper
- 2 tablespoons fresh cilantro, chopped

**Instructions**

1. Heat olive oil in a large skillet over medium heat.
2. Add diced onion and minced garlic. Sauté until the onion is translucent, about 3-4 minutes.
3. Add ground turkey and cook until no longer pink, about 5-6 minutes.
4. Add diced bell pepper and cook for an additional 3-4 minutes until tender.
5. Stir in cauliflower rice, ground cumin, ground turmeric, and ground black pepper. Cook for 5-6 minutes until cauliflower rice is tender.
6. Remove from heat and stir in fresh cilantro.
7. Serve warm.

**Nutrition Info per Serving**

- Calories: 230
- Protein: 25g
- Carbohydrates: 10g
- Fiber: 3g
- Sugars: 4g
- Fat: 10g
- Saturated Fat: 2g
- Sodium: 75mg

**Servings: 4**
**Cooking Time: 25 minutes**

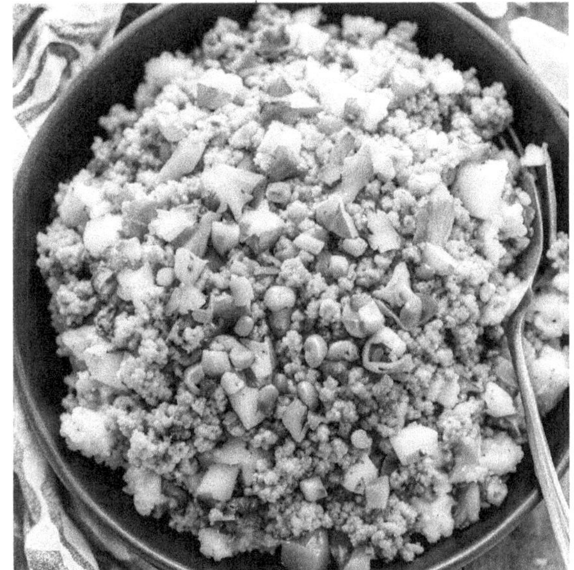

# Fish and Seafood Recipes

## 1. Grilled Salmon with Dill and Lemon

**Ingredients**

- 4 salmon fillets (about 6 ounces each)
- 2 tablespoons olive oil
- 2 tablespoons fresh dill, chopped
- 1 lemon, sliced
- 2 garlic cloves, minced
- 1/4 teaspoon ground black pepper

**Instructions**

1. Preheat the grill to medium-high heat.
2. In a small bowl, mix together olive oil, fresh dill, minced garlic, and ground black pepper.
3. Brush the salmon fillets with the olive oil mixture.
4. Place the salmon fillets on the grill and top each with a slice of lemon.
5. Grill for about 4-5 minutes per side, or until the salmon is opaque and flakes easily with a fork.
6. Remove from the grill and let rest for a few minutes before serving.

**Nutrition Info per Serving**

- Calories: 350
- Protein: 34g
- Carbohydrates: 2g
- Fiber: 0g
- Sugars: 0g
- Fat: 22g
- Saturated Fat: 3g
- Sodium: 85mg

**Servings: 4**
**Cooking Time: 15 minutes**

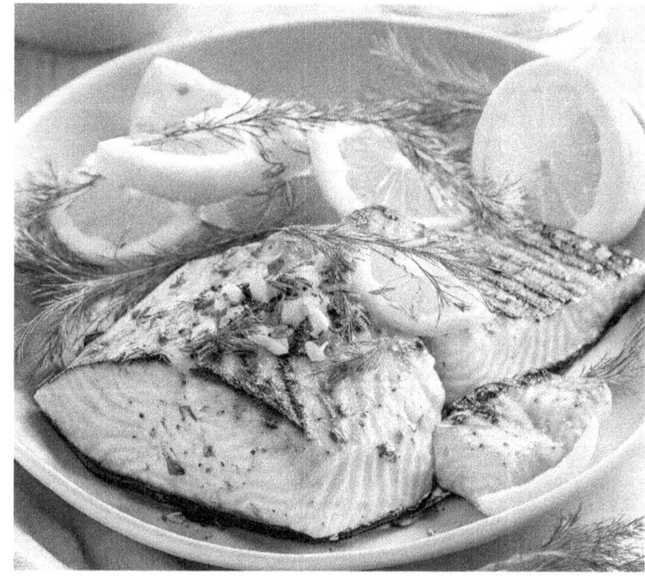

## 2. Baked Cod with Tomato and Basil

**Ingredients**

- 4 cod fillets (about 6 ounces each)
- 2 tablespoons olive oil
- 2 cups cherry tomatoes, halved
- 1/4 cup fresh basil, chopped
- 2 garlic cloves, minced
- 1/4 teaspoon ground black pepper

**Instructions**

1. Preheat the oven to 375°F (190°C).
2. In a baking dish, arrange the cod fillets.
3. In a bowl, mix together olive oil, cherry tomatoes, fresh basil, minced garlic, and ground black pepper.
4. Pour the tomato mixture over the cod fillets.
5. Bake in the preheated oven for 20-25 minutes, or until the fish is opaque and flakes easily with a fork.
6. Remove from the oven and let rest for a few minutes before serving.

**Nutrition Info per Serving**

- Calories: 200
- Protein: 35g
- Carbohydrates: 6g
- Fiber: 1g
- Sugars: 3g
- Fat: 6g
- Saturated Fat: 1g
- Sodium: 110mg

**Servings: 4**
**Cooking Time: 30 minutes**

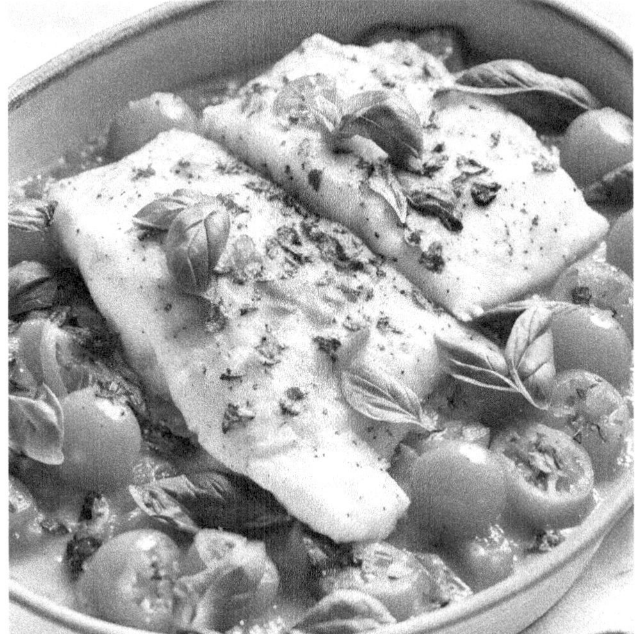

### 3. Pan-Seared Scallops with Garlic Spinach

**Ingredients**

- 1 pound large sea scallops
- 2 tablespoons olive oil, divided
- 2 garlic cloves, minced
- 4 cups fresh spinach
- 1 tablespoon lemon juice
- 1/4 teaspoon ground black pepper

**Instructions**

1. Heat 1 tablespoon of olive oil in a large skillet over medium-high heat.
2. Add the scallops to the skillet and sear for about 2-3 minutes on each side, until they are golden brown and opaque. Remove the scallops from the skillet and set aside.
3. In the same skillet, add the remaining olive oil and minced garlic. Sauté for 1-2 minutes until fragrant.
4. Add fresh spinach and cook until wilted, about 3-4 minutes.
5. Stir in lemon juice and ground black pepper.
6. Return the scallops to the skillet to warm through, about 1-2 minutes.
7. Remove from heat and serve immediately.

**Nutrition Info per Serving**

- Calories: 220
- Protein: 28g
- Carbohydrates: 5g
- Fiber: 2g
- Sugars: 1g
- Fat: 10g
- Saturated Fat: 1.5g
- Sodium: 180mg

**Servings: 4**
**Cooking Time: 20 minutes**

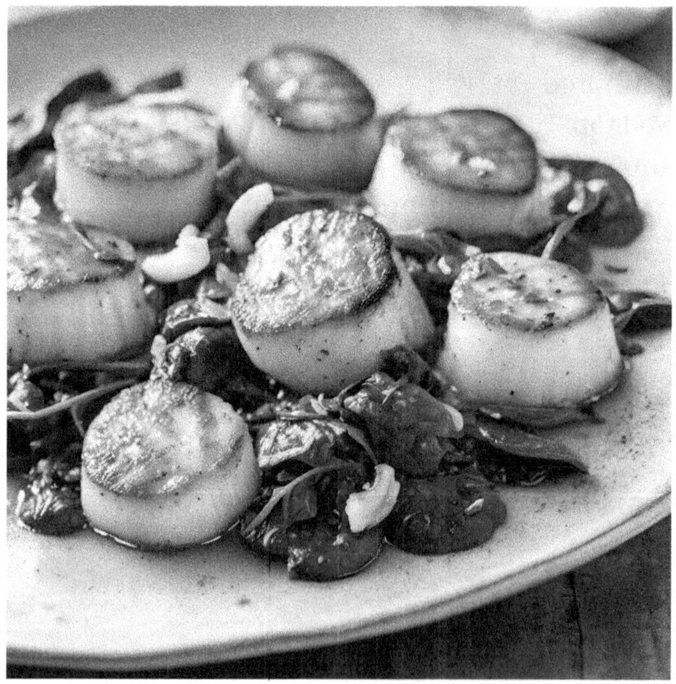

## 4. Shrimp and Avocado Salad

### Ingredients

- 1 pound large shrimp, peeled and deveined
- 2 tablespoons olive oil
- 1 avocado, diced
- 1 cup cherry tomatoes, halved
- 1/4 cup red onion, finely chopped
- 2 tablespoons fresh cilantro, chopped
- 1 tablespoon lime juice
- 1/4 teaspoon ground black pepper

### Instructions

1. Heat olive oil in a large skillet over medium-high heat.
2. Add the shrimp to the skillet and cook until pink and opaque, about 3-4 minutes per side. Remove from heat and let cool slightly.
3. In a large bowl, combine diced avocado, cherry tomatoes, red onion, and fresh cilantro.
4. Add the cooked shrimp to the bowl.
5. Drizzle with lime juice and sprinkle with ground black pepper.
6. Toss gently to combine.
7. Serve immediately.

### Nutrition Info per Serving

- Calories: 280
- Protein: 25g
- Carbohydrates: 10g
- Fiber: 5g
- Sugars: 3g
- Fat: 18g
- Saturated Fat: 2.5g
- Sodium: 210mg

**Servings: 4**
**Cooking Time: 15 minutes**

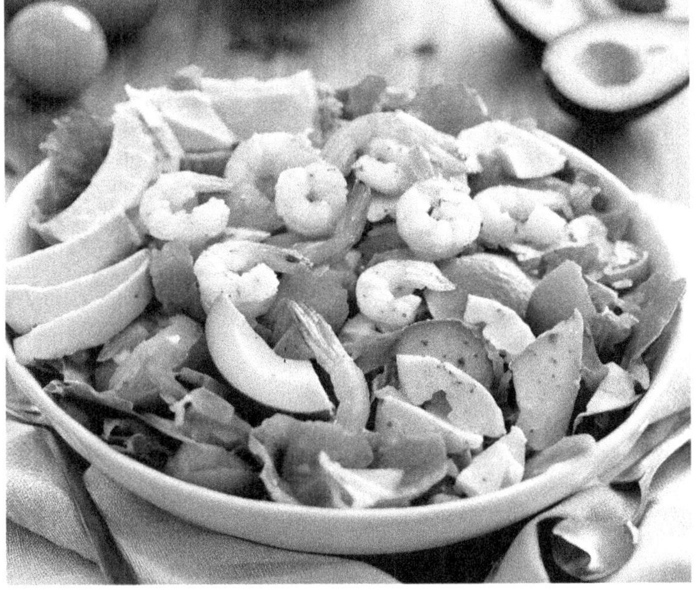

## 5. Poached Halibut with Fennel and Orange

**Ingredients**

- 4 halibut fillets (about 6 ounces each)
- 1 fennel bulb, thinly sliced
- 1 orange, thinly sliced
- 2 cups low-sodium vegetable broth
- 1 tablespoon olive oil
- 1 garlic clove, minced
- 1 tablespoon fresh dill, chopped
- 1/4 teaspoon ground black pepper

**Instructions**

1. In a large skillet, heat olive oil over medium heat. Add minced garlic and sauté for 1 minute until fragrant.
2. Add fennel slices to the skillet and cook for 3-4 minutes until slightly softened.
3. Pour in vegetable broth and bring to a simmer.
4. Arrange the halibut fillets on top of the fennel and add orange slices around the fish.
5. Cover the skillet and poach the fish for about 10-12 minutes, or until the fish is opaque and flakes easily with a fork.
6. Remove from heat and sprinkle with fresh dill and ground black pepper.
7. Serve warm.

**Nutrition Info per Serving**

- Calories: 250
- Protein: 30g
- Carbohydrates: 8g
- Fiber: 2g
- Sugars: 5g
- Fat: 10g
- Saturated Fat: 2g
- Sodium: 120mg

**Servings: 4**
**Cooking Time: 20 minutes**

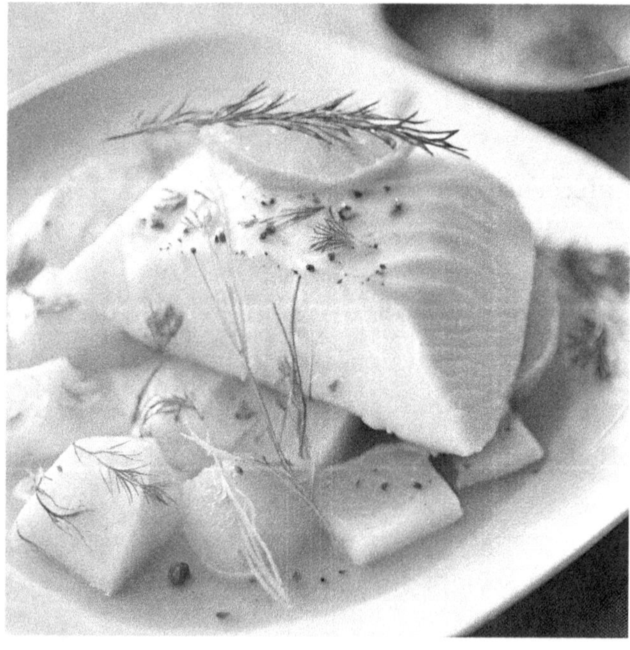

## 6. Tilapia with Mango Salsa

### Ingredients

- 4 tilapia fillets (about 6 ounces each)
- 1 tablespoon olive oil
- 1 ripe mango, diced
- 1/4 cup red bell pepper, diced
- 1/4 cup red onion, finely chopped
- 1 tablespoon fresh cilantro, chopped
- 1 tablespoon lime juice
- 1/4 teaspoon ground cumin

### Instructions

1. Preheat the oven to 375°F (190°C).
2. Brush tilapia fillets with olive oil and place them on a baking sheet lined with parchment paper.
3. Bake in the preheated oven for 15-20 minutes, or until the fish is opaque and flakes easily with a fork.
4. While the fish is baking, prepare the mango salsa by combining diced mango, red bell pepper, red onion, cilantro, lime juice, and ground cumin in a bowl. Mix well.
5. Remove tilapia from the oven and top with mango salsa.
6. Serve immediately.

### Nutrition Info per Serving

- Calories: 220
- Protein: 30g
- Carbohydrates: 12g
- Fiber: 2g
- Sugars: 9g
- Fat: 7g
- Saturated Fat: 1.5g
- Sodium: 90mg

**Servings: 4**
**Cooking Time: 25 minutes**

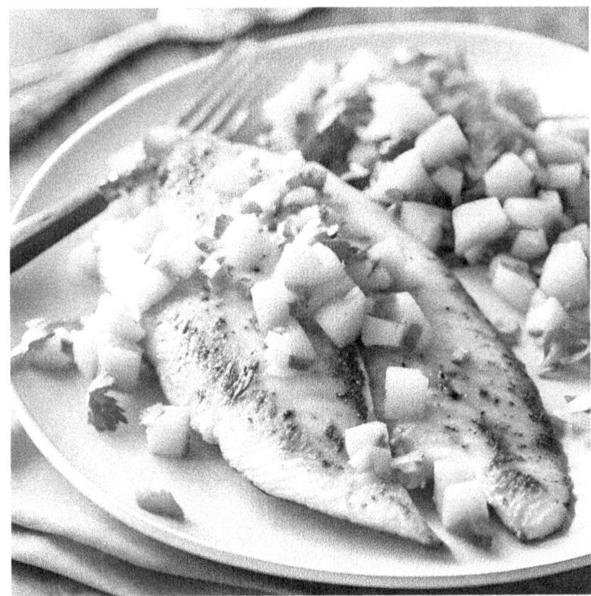

**7. Sea Bass en Papillote with Vegetables**

**Ingredients**

- 4 sea bass fillets (about 6 ounces each)
- 1 zucchini, julienned
- 1 carrot, julienned
- 1 red bell pepper, julienned
- 1 small leek, thinly sliced
- 2 tablespoons olive oil
- 1 lemon, thinly sliced
- 1 tablespoon fresh thyme leaves
- 1/4 teaspoon ground black pepper

**Instructions**

1. Preheat the oven to 375°F (190°C).
2. Cut 4 large pieces of parchment paper, each about 12 inches long.
3. In a bowl, toss together zucchini, carrot, bell pepper, leek, and 1 tablespoon of olive oil.
4. Place one sea bass fillet in the center of each parchment paper piece. Top with the mixed vegetables.
5. Drizzle each fillet with the remaining olive oil and sprinkle with thyme and ground black pepper.
6. Place lemon slices on top of the vegetables.
7. Fold the parchment paper over the fish and vegetables, crimping the edges to seal and create a packet.
8. Place the packets on a baking sheet and bake for 20-25 minutes, or until the fish is opaque and flakes easily with a fork.
9. Carefully open the packets and serve immediately.

**Nutrition Info per Serving**

- Calories: 280
- Protein: 32g
- Carbohydrates: 8g
- Fiber: 3g
- Sugars: 4g
- Fat: 14g
- Saturated Fat: 2g
- Sodium: 85mg

**Servings: 4**

**Cooking Time: 30 minutes**

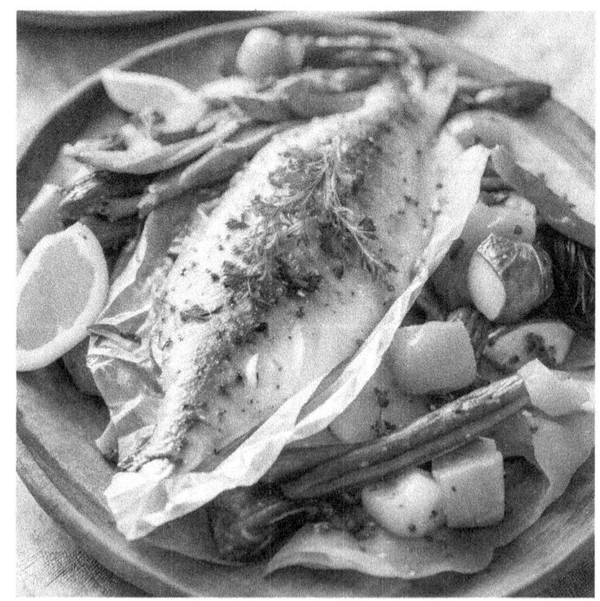

## 8. Shrimp Stir-Fry with Mixed Vegetables

### Ingredients

- 1 pound large shrimp, peeled and deveined
- 2 tablespoons olive oil
- 1 small onion, sliced
- 2 garlic cloves, minced
- 1 bell pepper, sliced
- 1 cup broccoli florets
- 1 cup snap peas
- 2 tablespoons low-sodium soy sauce
- 1 tablespoon fresh ginger, minced
- 1/4 teaspoon ground black pepper

### Instructions

1. Heat 1 tablespoon of olive oil in a large skillet or wok over medium-high heat.
2. Add the shrimp and cook until pink and opaque, about 3-4 minutes. Remove the shrimp from the skillet and set aside.
3. In the same skillet, add the remaining olive oil. Add sliced onion and minced garlic, and sauté for 2-3 minutes until the onion is translucent.
4. Add bell pepper, broccoli, and snap peas to the skillet. Stir-fry for about 5-6 minutes until the vegetables are tender but still crisp.
5. Stir in soy sauce, minced ginger, and ground black pepper.
6. Return the shrimp to the skillet and toss to combine.
7. Cook for an additional 1-2 minutes until everything is heated through.
8. Remove from heat and serve immediately.

### Nutrition Info per Serving

- Calories: 220
- Protein: 25g
- Carbohydrates: 10g
- Fiber: 3g
- Sugars: 4g
- Fat: 10g
- Saturated Fat: 1.5g
- Sodium: 340mg

**Servings: 4**

**Cooking Time: 20 minutes**

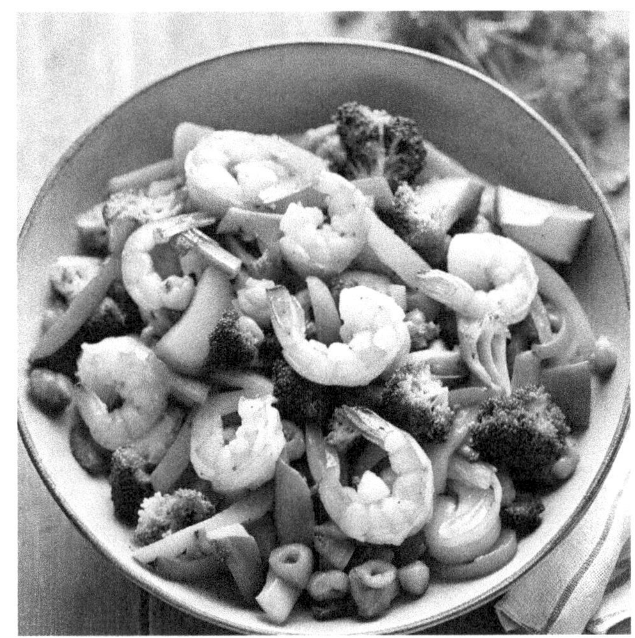

## 9. Clam Chowder with Sweet Potatoes

### Ingredients

- 2 tablespoons olive oil
- 1 small onion, diced
- 2 garlic cloves, minced
- 2 cups sweet potatoes, peeled and diced
- 2 cups low-sodium vegetable broth
- 1 cup unsweetened almond milk
- 1 pound clams, cleaned
- 1 teaspoon dried thyme
- 1/4 teaspoon ground black pepper
- 1 tablespoon fresh parsley, chopped

### Instructions

1. Heat olive oil in a large pot over medium heat.
2. Add diced onion and minced garlic. Sauté until the onion is translucent, about 3-4 minutes.
3. Add diced sweet potatoes to the pot and cook for an additional 5 minutes.
4. Pour in vegetable broth and bring to a boil.
5. Reduce heat to a simmer and add dried thyme and ground black pepper. Cook until the sweet potatoes are tender, about 10-15 minutes.
6. Stir in almond milk and clams. Cover and cook until the clams open, about 5-7 minutes. Discard any clams that do not open.
7. Remove from heat and sprinkle with fresh parsley.
8. Serve warm.

### Nutrition Info per Serving

- Calories: 300
- Protein: 20g
- Carbohydrates: 30g
- Fiber: 5g
- Sugars: 8g
- Fat: 10g
- Saturated Fat: 1.5g
- Sodium: 220mg

**Servings: 4**
**Cooking Time: 35 minutes**

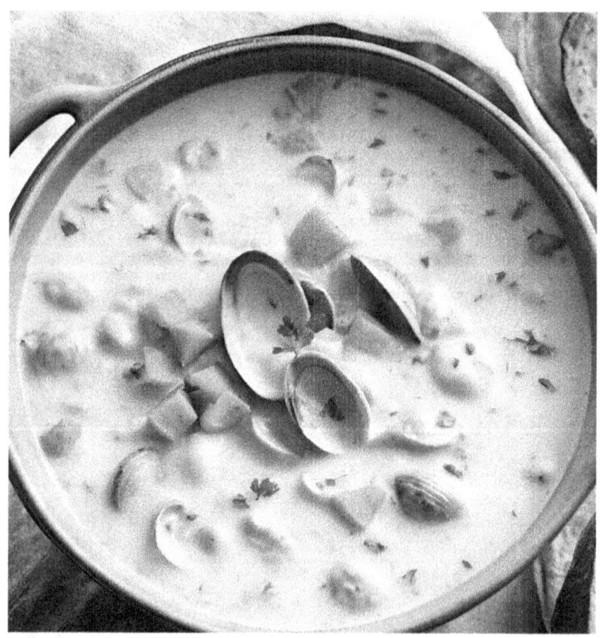

## 10. Mackerel Salad with Mustard Vinaigrette

**Ingredients**

- 4 mackerel fillets (about 6 ounces each)
- 1 tablespoon olive oil
- 6 cups mixed greens (arugula, spinach, and lettuce)
- 1 cup cherry tomatoes, halved
- 1 small cucumber, sliced
- 1/4 cup red onion, thinly sliced
- 1 tablespoon fresh parsley, chopped

Mustard Vinaigrette:

- 2 tablespoons Dijon mustard
- 1 tablespoon apple cider vinegar
- 3 tablespoons olive oil
- 1 teaspoon honey
- 1/4 teaspoon ground black pepper

**Instructions**

1. Preheat the grill to medium-high heat.
2. Brush the mackerel fillets with olive oil and grill for about 4-5 minutes on each side, until cooked through and flaky. Remove from the grill and let cool slightly.
3. In a large bowl, combine mixed greens, cherry tomatoes, cucumber, and red onion.
4. In a small bowl, whisk together Dijon mustard, apple cider vinegar, olive oil, honey, and ground black pepper to make the vinaigrette.
5. Pour the vinaigrette over the salad and toss to combine.
6. Flake the grilled mackerel over the salad and sprinkle with fresh parsley.
7. Serve immediately.

**Nutrition Info per Serving**

- Calories: 350
- Protein: 30g
- Carbohydrates: 10g
- Fiber: 3g
- Sugars: 5g
- Fat: 20g
- Saturated Fat: 3.5g
- Sodium: 150mg

**Servings: 4**
**Cooking Time: 20 minutes**

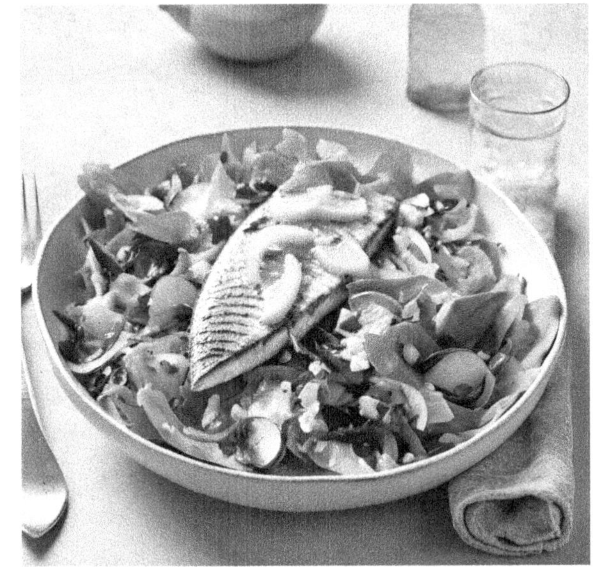

## 11. Baked Trout with Almonds

### Ingredients

- 4 trout fillets (about 6 ounces each)
- 2 tablespoons olive oil
- 1/2 cup sliced almonds
- 1 lemon, thinly sliced
- 1 garlic clove, minced
- 1 tablespoon fresh dill, chopped
- 1/4 teaspoon ground black pepper

### Instructions

1. Preheat the oven to 375°F (190°C).
2. Place the trout fillets in a baking dish.
3. In a small bowl, mix together olive oil, minced garlic, and ground black pepper. Brush this mixture over the trout fillets.
4. Sprinkle sliced almonds over the fillets and arrange lemon slices on top.
5. Bake in the preheated oven for 20-25 minutes, or until the trout is opaque and flakes easily with a fork.
6. Remove from the oven and sprinkle with fresh dill.
7. Serve warm.

### Nutrition Info per Serving

- Calories: 350
- Protein: 30g
- Carbohydrates: 6g
- Fiber: 2g
- Sugars: 2g
- Fat: 22g
- Saturated Fat: 3g
- Sodium: 100mg

**Servings: 4**
**Cooking Time: 30 minutes**

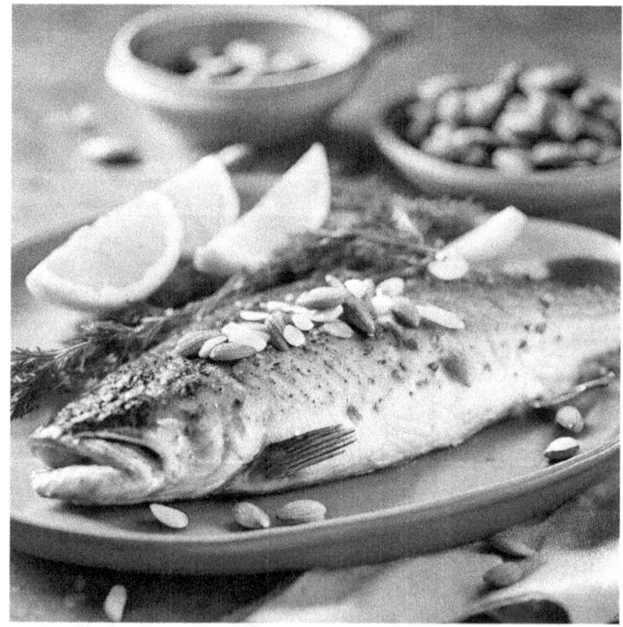

## 12. Tuna Steak with Olive Tapenade

### Ingredients

- 4 tuna steaks (about 6 ounces each)
- 2 tablespoons olive oil
- 1 tablespoon lemon juice
- 1/2 cup mixed olives, pitted and chopped
- 1 garlic clove, minced
- 1 tablespoon capers, drained
- 1 tablespoon fresh parsley, chopped
- 1/4 teaspoon ground black pepper

### Instructions

1. Preheat the grill to medium-high heat.
2. Brush the tuna steaks with olive oil and lemon juice.
3. Grill the tuna steaks for about 3-4 minutes on each side, until seared on the outside but still pink in the center. Remove from the grill and let rest for a few minutes.
4. In a small bowl, combine chopped olives, minced garlic, capers, fresh parsley, and ground black pepper to make the olive tapenade.
5. Top each tuna steak with a generous spoonful of olive tapenade.
6. Serve immediately.

### Nutrition Info per Serving

- Calories: 320
- Protein: 35g
- Carbohydrates: 3g
- Fiber: 1g
- Sugars: 0g
- Fat: 20g
- Saturated Fat: 3g
- Sodium: 250mg

**Servings: 4**
**Cooking Time: 20 minutes**

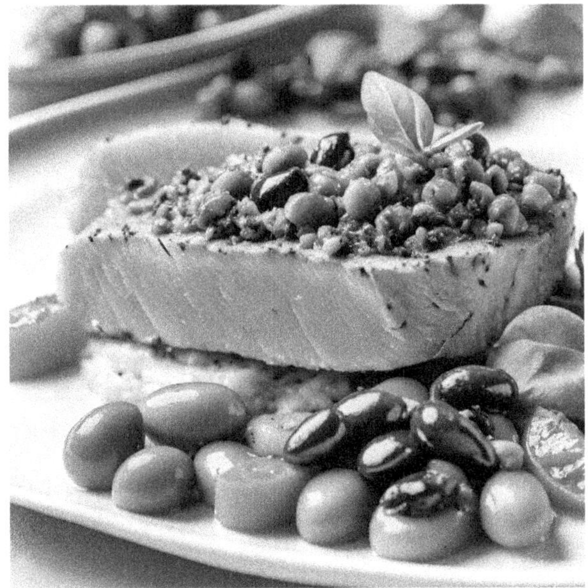

## 13. Haddock in Parsley Sauce

### Ingredients

- 4 haddock fillets (about 6 ounces each)
- 2 tablespoons olive oil
- 1 cup low-sodium vegetable broth
- 1/2 cup unsweetened almond milk
- 2 tablespoons whole wheat flour
- 2 tablespoons fresh parsley, chopped
- 1 lemon, zested and juiced
- 1/4 teaspoon ground black pepper

### Instructions

1. Preheat the oven to 375°F (190°C).
2. Heat olive oil in a skillet over medium heat. Add whole wheat flour and cook for 1-2 minutes to form a roux.
3. Gradually whisk in vegetable broth and almond milk, stirring constantly to avoid lumps. Bring to a simmer.
4. Add lemon zest, lemon juice, and ground black pepper. Simmer for 5-7 minutes until the sauce thickens.
5. Place the haddock fillets in a baking dish and pour the parsley sauce over them.
6. Bake in the preheated oven for 20-25 minutes, or until the fish is opaque and flakes easily with a fork.
7. Remove from the oven and sprinkle with fresh parsley.
8. Serve warm.

### Nutrition Info per Serving

- Calories: 240
- Protein: 30g
- Carbohydrates: 6g
- Fiber: 1g
- Sugars: 1g
- Fat: 10g
- Saturated Fat: 1.5g
- Sodium: 150mg

**Servings: 4**

**Cooking Time: 30 minutes**

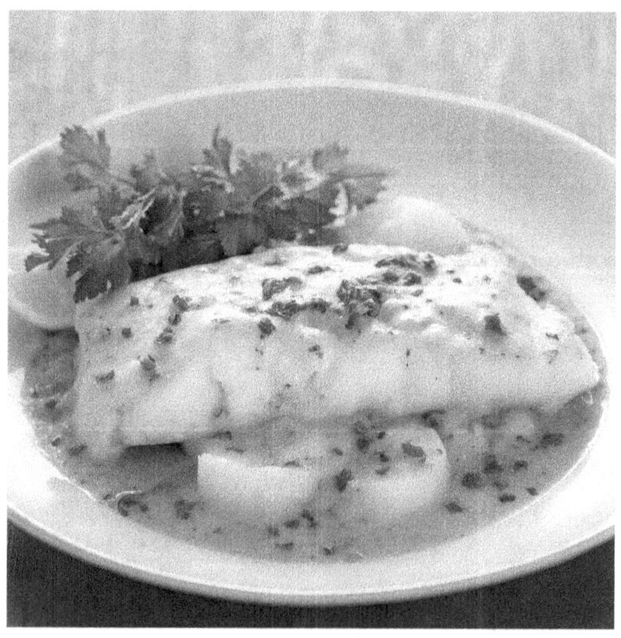

## 14. Seafood Paella with Brown Rice

### Ingredients

- 1 cup brown rice
- 2 tablespoons olive oil
- 1 small onion, diced
- 2 garlic cloves, minced
- 1 red bell pepper, diced
- 1 cup diced tomatoes
- 1 teaspoon smoked paprika
- 1/2 teaspoon ground turmeric
- 4 cups low-sodium vegetable broth
- 1/2 pound shrimp, peeled and deveined
- 1/2 pound mussels, cleaned
- 1/2 pound squid rings
- 1/2 cup frozen peas
- 1 tablespoon fresh parsley, chopped
- 1 lemon, cut into wedges

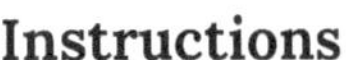

### Instructions

1. Heat olive oil in a large skillet or paella pan over medium heat.
2. Add diced onion, minced garlic, and red bell pepper. Sauté for 3-4 minutes until the onion is translucent.
3. Add brown rice, diced tomatoes, smoked paprika, and ground turmeric. Stir well to combine.
4. Pour in vegetable broth and bring to a boil.
5. Reduce heat to a simmer and cook for 30-35 minutes, or until the rice is tender and most of the liquid is absorbed.
6. Add shrimp, mussels, squid rings, and frozen peas to the pan. Cook for an additional 10 minutes until the seafood is cooked through and the mussels have opened.
7. Remove from heat and sprinkle with fresh parsley.
8. Serve warm with lemon wedges.

### Nutrition Info per Serving

- Calories: 350
- Protein: 28g
- Carbohydrates: 35g
- Fiber: 5g
- Sugars: 6g
- Fat: 12g
- Saturated Fat: 2g
- Sodium: 220mg

**Servings: 4**
**Cooking Time: 50 minutes**

**15. Steamed Mussels in White Wine and Garlic**
**Ingredients**

- 2 pounds mussels, cleaned
- 2 tablespoons olive oil
- 4 garlic cloves, minced
- 1 cup dry white wine
- 1/4 cup fresh parsley, chopped
- 1 lemon, juiced
- 1/4 teaspoon ground black pepper

**Instructions**

1. Heat olive oil in a large pot over medium heat.
2. Add minced garlic and sauté for 1-2 minutes until fragrant.
3. Pour in the white wine and bring to a simmer.
4. Add the cleaned mussels to the pot and cover with a lid.
5. Steam the mussels for 5-7 minutes, or until they open. Discard any mussels that do not open.
6. Remove from heat and stir in lemon juice, chopped parsley, and ground black pepper.
7. Serve immediately with the broth.

**Nutrition Info per Serving**

- Calories: 250
- Protein: 20g
- Carbohydrates: 8g
- Fiber: 1g
- Sugars: 2g
- Fat: 10g
- Saturated Fat: 1.5g
- Sodium: 320mg

**Servings: 4**
**Cooking Time: 20 minutes**

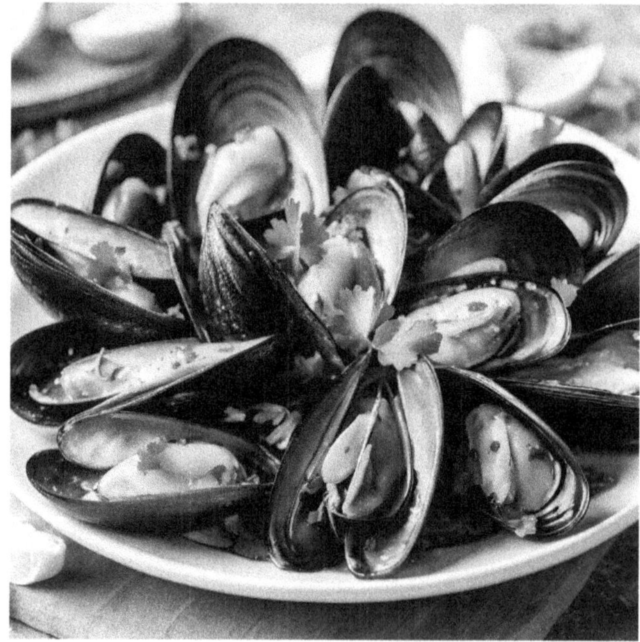

## 16. Teriyaki Glazed Salmon

### Ingredients

- 4 salmon fillets (about 6 ounces each)
- 1/4 cup low-sodium soy sauce
- 2 tablespoons honey
- 2 tablespoons rice vinegar
- 1 garlic clove, minced
- 1 teaspoon fresh ginger, grated
- 1 tablespoon olive oil
- 1 tablespoon sesame seeds
- 2 tablespoons green onions, chopped

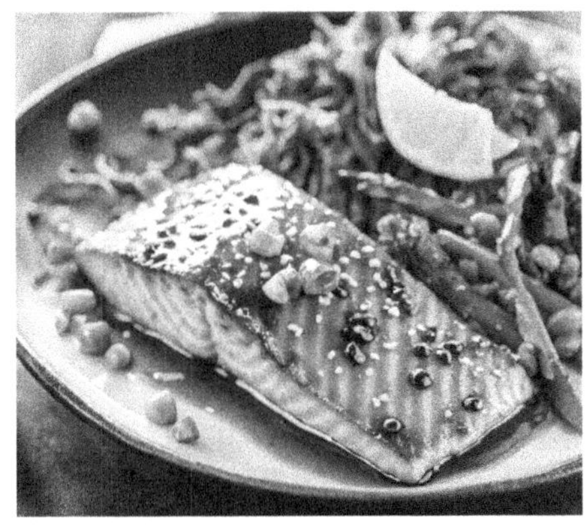

### Instructions

1. In a small bowl, whisk together soy sauce, honey, rice vinegar, minced garlic, and grated ginger.
2. Place the salmon fillets in a shallow dish and pour the marinade over them. Let marinate for at least 30 minutes in the refrigerator.
3. Preheat the oven to 375°F (190°C).
4. Heat olive oil in a large oven-safe skillet over medium heat.
5. Remove the salmon from the marinade and place in the skillet, skin-side down. Reserve the marinade.
6. Sear the salmon for 2-3 minutes until the skin is crispy.
7. Pour the reserved marinade over the salmon and transfer the skillet to the preheated oven.
8. Bake for 10-12 minutes, or until the salmon is cooked through and flakes easily with a fork.
9. Remove from the oven and sprinkle with sesame seeds and chopped green onions.
10. Serve immediately.

### Nutrition Info per Serving

- Calories: 320
- Protein: 34g
- Carbohydrates: 12g
- Fiber: 0g
- Sugars: 9g
- Fat: 16g
- Saturated Fat: 2.5g
- Sodium: 500mg

**Servings: 4**
**Cooking Time: 40 minutes (including marinating time)**

## 17. Orange Ginger Glazed Salmon

**Ingredients**

- 4 salmon fillets (about 6 ounces each)
- 1/4 cup orange juice
- 2 tablespoons honey
- 1 tablespoon fresh ginger, grated
- 2 garlic cloves, minced
- 1 tablespoon olive oil
- 1 orange, zested
- 1 tablespoon fresh cilantro, chopped

**Instructions**

1. In a small bowl, whisk together orange juice, honey, grated ginger, minced garlic, and orange zest.
2. Place the salmon fillets in a shallow dish and pour the marinade over them. Let marinate for at least 30 minutes in the refrigerator.
3. Preheat the oven to 375°F (190°C).
4. Heat olive oil in a large oven-safe skillet over medium heat.
5. Remove the salmon from the marinade and place in the skillet, skin-side down. Reserve the marinade.
6. Sear the salmon for 2-3 minutes until the skin is crispy.
7. Pour the reserved marinade over the salmon and transfer the skillet to the preheated oven.
8. Bake for 10-12 minutes, or until the salmon is cooked through and flakes easily with a fork.
9. Remove from the oven and sprinkle with chopped cilantro.
10. Serve immediately.

**Nutrition Info per Serving**

- Calories: 310
- Protein: 34g
- Carbohydrates: 11g
- Fiber: 0g
- Sugars: 9g
- Fat: 16g
- Saturated Fat: 2.5g
- Sodium: 85mg

**Servings: 4**

**Cooking Time: 40 minutes (including marinating time)**

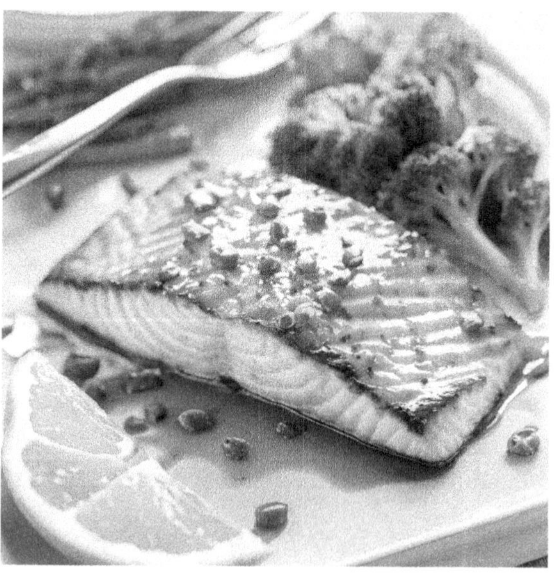

## 18. Sardine and Tomato Bruschetta

### Ingredients

- 1 can sardines in olive oil, drained and flaked
- 1 cup cherry tomatoes, diced
- 1 small red onion, finely chopped
- 2 tablespoons fresh basil, chopped
- 1 tablespoon balsamic vinegar
- 1 garlic clove, minced
- 1 baguette, sliced and toasted
- 1 tablespoon olive oil
- 1/4 teaspoon ground black pepper

### Instructions

1. In a bowl, combine flaked sardines, diced cherry tomatoes, finely chopped red onion, chopped basil, balsamic vinegar, minced garlic, and ground black pepper. Mix well.
2. Brush the baguette slices with olive oil and toast until golden brown.
3. Spoon the sardine and tomato mixture onto the toasted baguette slices.
4. Serve immediately.

### Nutrition Info per Serving

- Calories: 180
- Protein: 10g
- Carbohydrates: 15g
- Fiber: 2g
- Sugars: 3g
- Fat: 9g
- Saturated Fat: 1.5g
- Sodium: 230mg

**Servings: 4**
**Cooking Time: 15 minutes**

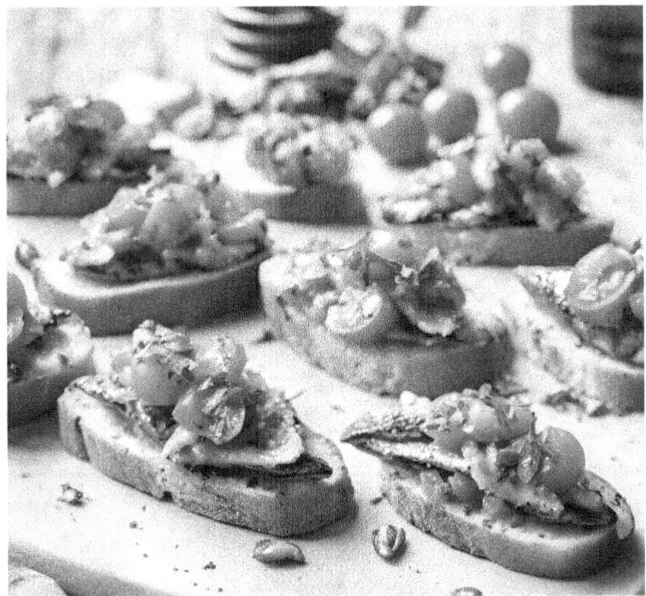

## 19. Pan-Seared Tuna with Avocado Salad

**Ingredients**

- 4 tuna steaks (about 6 ounces each)
- 2 tablespoons olive oil
- 1 tablespoon lemon juice
- 1 teaspoon fresh ginger, grated
- 1 avocado, diced
- 1 cup cherry tomatoes, halved
- 1/4 cup red onion, finely chopped
- 2 tablespoons fresh cilantro, chopped
- 1 tablespoon lime juice
- 1/4 teaspoon ground cumin

**Instructions**

1. In a small bowl, mix together olive oil, lemon juice, and grated ginger.
2. Brush the tuna steaks with the olive oil mixture and let marinate for 10-15 minutes.
3. In another bowl, combine diced avocado, cherry tomatoes, red onion, cilantro, lime juice, and ground cumin. Mix well to make the avocado salad.
4. Heat a non-stick skillet over medium-high heat.
5. Sear the tuna steaks for 2-3 minutes on each side, until they are cooked to your desired doneness.
6. Remove from heat and let rest for a few minutes.
7. Serve the tuna steaks with the avocado salad on the side.

**Nutrition Info per Serving**

- Calories: 350
- Protein: 35g
- Carbohydrates: 8g
- Fiber: 4g
- Sugars: 2g
- Fat: 20g
- Saturated Fat: 3g
- Sodium: 90mg

**Servings: 4**
**Cooking Time: 20 minutes**

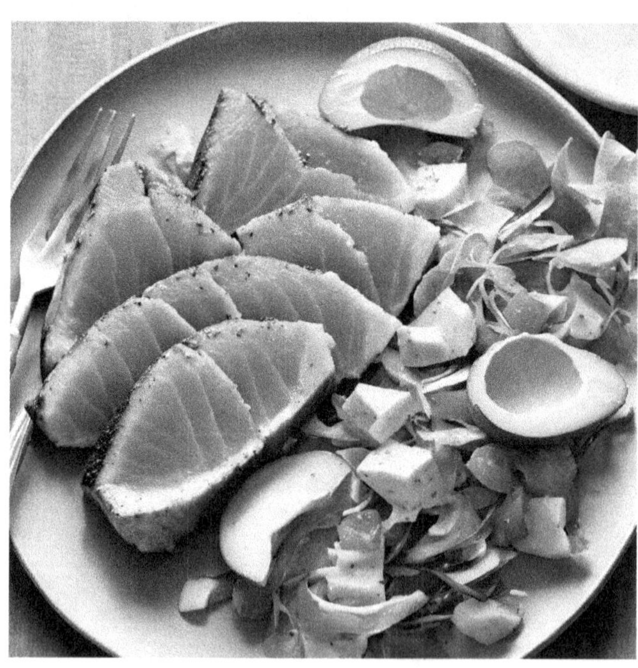

## 20. Herb-Crusted Halibut with Roasted Vegetables

### Ingredients

- 4 halibut fillets (about 6 ounces each)
- 1/4 cup whole wheat breadcrumbs
- 2 tablespoons fresh parsley, chopped
- 1 tablespoon fresh thyme, chopped
- 2 garlic cloves, minced
- 2 tablespoons olive oil
- 2 cups baby carrots
- 2 cups Brussels sprouts, halved
- 1 red bell pepper, sliced
- 1 tablespoon lemon juice

### Instructions

1. Preheat the oven to 375°F (190°C).
2. In a small bowl, mix together breadcrumbs, parsley, thyme, minced garlic, and 1 tablespoon of olive oil.
3. Place the halibut fillets on a baking sheet lined with parchment paper. Press the breadcrumb mixture onto the top of each fillet.
4. In a large bowl, toss baby carrots, Brussels sprouts, and red bell pepper with the remaining olive oil and lemon juice.
5. Spread the vegetables around the halibut fillets on the baking sheet.
6. Bake in the preheated oven for 20-25 minutes, or until the halibut is opaque and flakes easily with a fork and the vegetables are tender.
7. Remove from the oven and serve warm.

### Nutrition Info per Serving

- Calories: 300
- Protein: 30g
- Carbohydrates: 18g
- Fiber: 6g
- Sugars: 6g
- Fat: 12g
- Saturated Fat: 2g
- Sodium: 150mg

**Servings: 4**
**Cooking Time: 30 minutes**

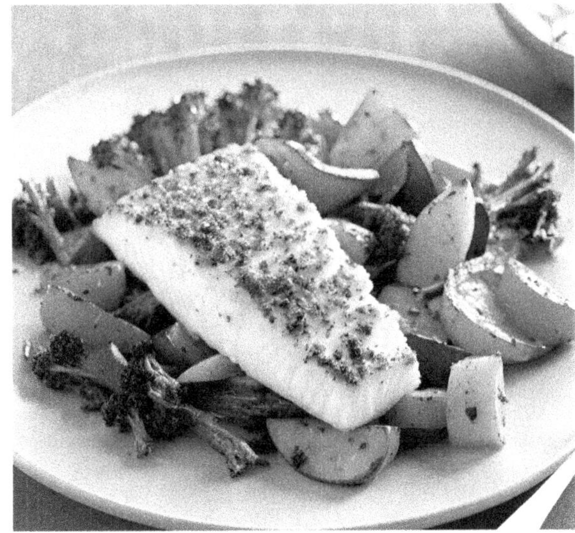

## 21. Baked Lemon Sole with Capers

### Ingredients

- 4 sole fillets (about 6 ounces each)
- 2 tablespoons olive oil
- 1 lemon, zested and juiced
- 2 tablespoons capers, drained
- 2 garlic cloves, minced
- 1 tablespoon fresh dill, chopped
- 1/4 teaspoon ground black pepper

### Instructions

1. Preheat the oven to 375°F (190°C).
2. Place the sole fillets in a baking dish.
3. In a small bowl, mix together olive oil, lemon zest, lemon juice, capers, minced garlic, and ground black pepper.
4. Pour the lemon mixture over the sole fillets.
5. Bake in the preheated oven for 15-20 minutes, or until the fish is opaque and flakes easily with a fork.
6. Remove from the oven and sprinkle with fresh dill.
7. Serve immediately.

### Nutrition Info per Serving

- Calories: 220
- Protein: 28g
- Carbohydrates: 4g
- Fiber: 1g
- Sugars: 1g
- Fat: 10g
- Saturated Fat: 1.5g
- Sodium: 210mg

**Servings: 4**

**Cooking Time: 20 minutes**

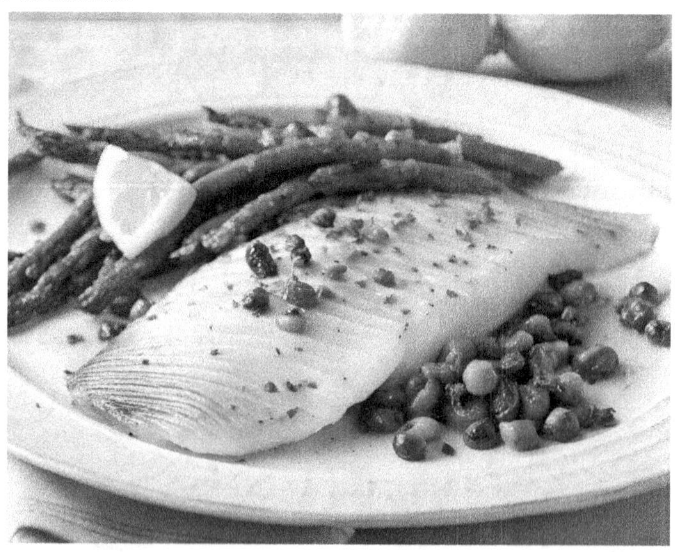

## 22. Spiced Cod with Lentils

**Ingredients**

- 4 cod fillets (about 6 ounces each)
- 2 tablespoons olive oil, divided
- 1 teaspoon ground cumin
- 1/2 teaspoon ground turmeric
- 1/2 teaspoon ground coriander
- 1 cup dried green or brown lentils, rinsed
- 1 small onion, diced
- 2 garlic cloves, minced
- 1 carrot, diced
- 4 cups low-sodium vegetable broth
- 1 tablespoon fresh parsley, chopped

**Instructions**

1. In a small bowl, mix together ground cumin, turmeric, and coriander.
2. Rub the spice mixture onto the cod fillets.
3. Heat 1 tablespoon of olive oil in a large skillet over medium heat. Add the spiced cod fillets and cook for 3-4 minutes on each side, until the fish is opaque and flakes easily with a fork. Remove from heat and set aside.
4. In a large pot, heat the remaining olive oil over medium heat. Add diced onion, minced garlic, and diced carrot. Sauté for 5-6 minutes until the vegetables are tender.
5. Add the lentils and vegetable broth to the pot. Bring to a boil, then reduce heat and simmer for 20-25 minutes, or until the lentils are tender and most of the liquid is absorbed.
6. Remove from heat and stir in fresh parsley.
7. Serve the spiced cod fillets over a bed of lentils.

**Nutrition Info per Serving**

- Calories: 320
- Protein: 32g
- Carbohydrates: 28g
- Fiber: 9g
- Sugars: 4g
- Fat: 10g
- Saturated Fat: 1.5g
- Sodium: 200mg

**Servings: 4**
**Cooking Time: 40 minutes**

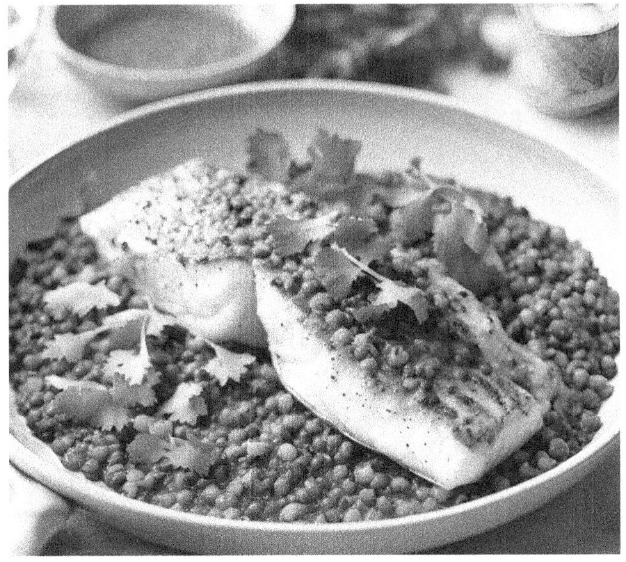

# Vegetables

**1. Roasted Brussels Sprouts with Garlic**
**Ingredients**
- 1 pound Brussels sprouts, trimmed and halved
- 3 garlic cloves, minced
- 2 tablespoons olive oil
- 1 tablespoon balsamic vinegar
- 1/4 teaspoon ground black pepper

Instructions
1. Preheat the oven to 400°F (200°C).
2. In a large bowl, combine Brussels sprouts, minced garlic, olive oil, balsamic vinegar, and ground black pepper. Toss to coat evenly.
3. Spread the Brussels sprouts mixture on a baking sheet in a single layer.
4. Roast in the preheated oven for 20-25 minutes, stirring halfway through, until the Brussels sprouts are tender and golden brown.
5. Remove from the oven and serve warm.

**Nutrition Info per Serving**
- Calories: 120
- Protein: 4g
- Carbohydrates: 12g
- Fiber: 4g
- Sugars: 3g
- Fat: 8g
- Saturated Fat: 1g
- Sodium: 50mg

**Servings: 4**
**Cooking Time: 30 minutes**

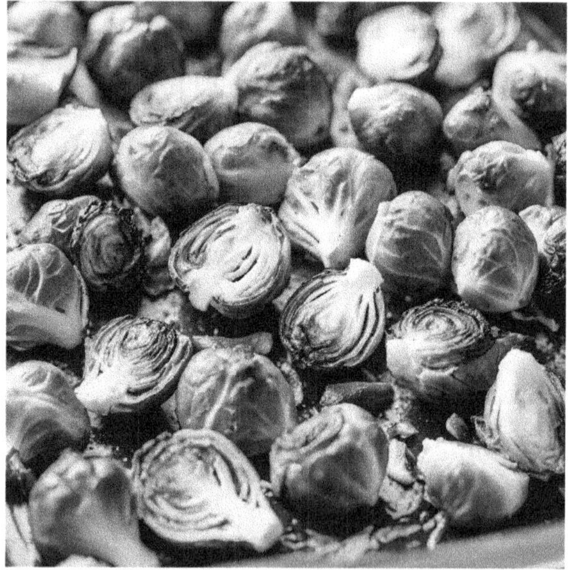

## 2. Spicy Kale and Coconut Stir Fry

**Ingredients**

- 1 bunch kale, stems removed and leaves chopped
- 1 tablespoon coconut oil
- 1 small onion, sliced
- 2 garlic cloves, minced
- 1 red bell pepper, sliced
- 1/2 teaspoon ground turmeric
- 1/4 teaspoon ground cumin
- 1/4 teaspoon ground chili flakes
- 1/4 cup unsweetened coconut flakes

**Instructions**

1. Heat coconut oil in a large skillet over medium heat.
2. Add sliced onion and minced garlic. Sauté for 3-4 minutes until the onion is translucent.
3. Add sliced red bell pepper and cook for another 2-3 minutes until slightly tender.
4. Add chopped kale, ground turmeric, ground cumin, and ground chili flakes. Stir well to combine.
5. Cook for 5-7 minutes, stirring occasionally, until the kale is wilted and tender.
6. Stir in unsweetened coconut flakes and cook for an additional 1-2 minutes.
7. Remove from heat and serve warm.

**Nutrition Info per Serving**

- Calories: 140
- Protein: 3g
- Carbohydrates: 10g
- Fiber: 4g
- Sugars: 2g
- Fat: 10g
- Saturated Fat: 8g
- Sodium: 40mg

**Servings: 4**
**Cooking Time: 20 minutes**

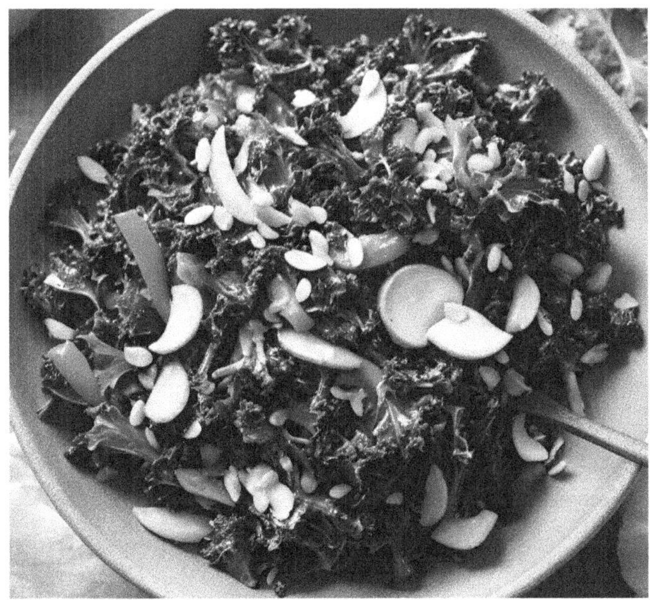

## 3. Baked Sweet Potato Fries

**Ingredients**

- 2 large sweet potatoes, peeled and cut into fries
- 2 tablespoons olive oil
- 1/2 teaspoon ground paprika
- 1/4 teaspoon ground cumin
- 1/4 teaspoon ground black pepper

**Instructions**

1. Preheat the oven to 425°F (220°C).
2. In a large bowl, combine sweet potato fries, olive oil, ground paprika, ground cumin, and ground black pepper. Toss to coat evenly.
3. Spread the sweet potato fries on a baking sheet in a single layer.
4. Bake in the preheated oven for 25-30 minutes, flipping halfway through, until the fries are crispy and golden brown.
5. Remove from the oven and serve warm.

**Nutrition Info per Serving**

- Calories: 180
- Protein: 2g
- Carbohydrates: 28g
- Fiber: 4g
- Sugars: 6g
- Fat: 7g
- Saturated Fat: 1g
- Sodium: 50mg

**Servings: 4**
**Cooking Time: 30 minutes**

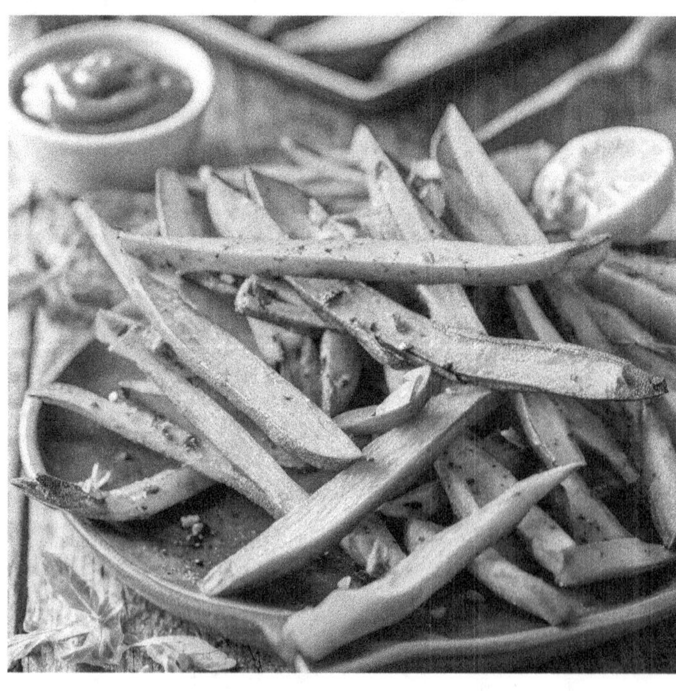

## 4. Zucchini Noodles with Pesto

### Ingredients

- 4 medium zucchinis, spiralized
- 2 cups fresh basil leaves
- 1/4 cup pine nuts
- 2 garlic cloves
- 1/4 cup olive oil
- 1/4 cup nutritional yeast
- 1 tablespoon lemon juice
- 1/4 teaspoon ground black pepper

### Instructions

1. In a food processor, combine fresh basil leaves, pine nuts, garlic cloves, olive oil, nutritional yeast, lemon juice, and ground black pepper. Process until smooth to make the pesto sauce.
2. In a large skillet, heat a small amount of olive oil over medium heat.
3. Add the spiralized zucchini noodles and cook for 2-3 minutes until slightly tender.
4. Remove from heat and toss the zucchini noodles with the pesto sauce until evenly coated.
5. Serve immediately.

### Nutrition Info per Serving

- Calories: 180
- Protein: 4g
- Carbohydrates: 6g
- Fiber: 2g
- Sugars: 4g
- Fat: 16g
- Saturated Fat: 2.5g
- Sodium: 50mg

**Servings: 4**
**Cooking Time: 15 minutes**

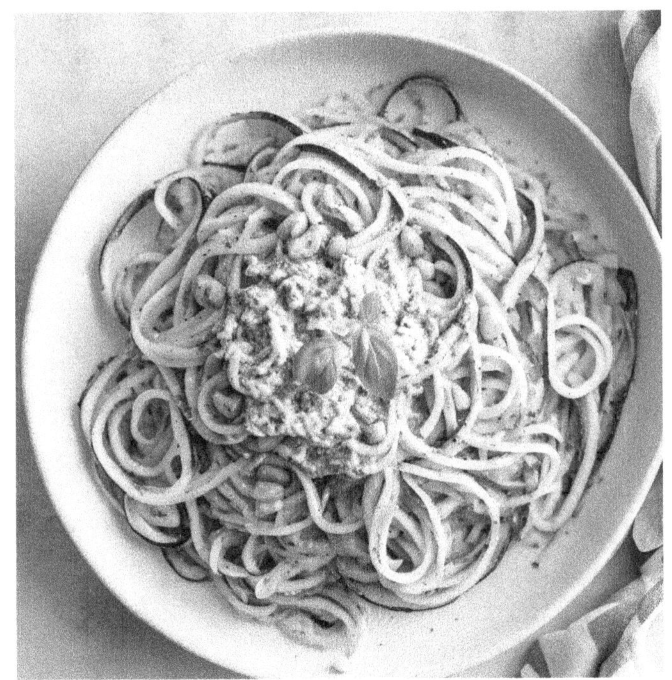

## 5. Stuffed Bell Peppers with Quinoa

**Ingredients**

- 4 large bell peppers, tops cut off and seeds removed
- 1 cup quinoa, rinsed
- 2 cups low-sodium vegetable broth
- 1 small onion, diced
- 2 garlic cloves, minced
- 1 cup diced tomatoes
- 1 cup black beans, drained and rinsed
- 1 teaspoon ground cumin
- 1 teaspoon ground paprika
- 1/4 teaspoon ground black pepper
- 1 tablespoon olive oil
- 1/4 cup fresh cilantro, chopped

**Instructions**

1. Preheat the oven to 375°F (190°C).
2. In a medium pot, bring vegetable broth to a boil. Add quinoa, reduce heat to low, cover, and simmer for 15 minutes or until the quinoa is cooked and the liquid is absorbed.
3. In a large skillet, heat olive oil over medium heat. Add diced onion and minced garlic, and sauté for 3-4 minutes until the onion is translucent.
4. Add diced tomatoes, black beans, cooked quinoa, ground cumin, ground paprika, and ground black pepper to the skillet. Stir well to combine and cook for an additional 5 minutes.
5. Stuff the bell peppers with the quinoa mixture and place them in a baking dish.
6. Cover with foil and bake in the preheated oven for 25-30 minutes, until the bell peppers are tender.
7. Remove from the oven and sprinkle with fresh cilantro.
8. Serve warm.

**Nutrition Info per Serving**

- Calories: 220
- Protein: 8g
- Carbohydrates: 38g
- Fiber: 8g
- Sugars: 8g
- Fat: 5g
- Saturated Fat: 0.5g
- Sodium: 120mg

**Servings: 4**

**Cooking Time: 40 minutes**

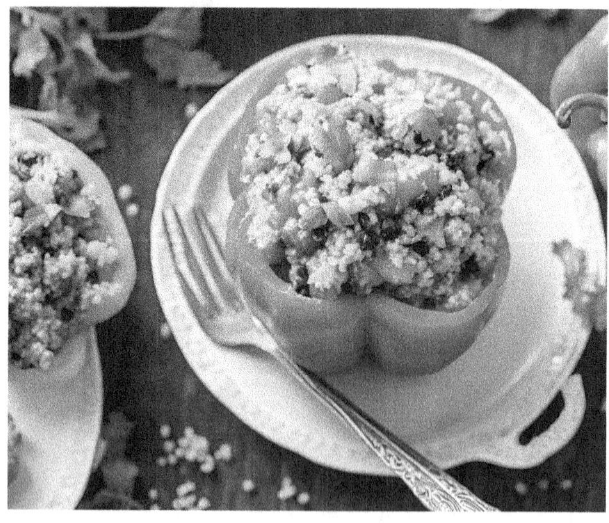

## 6. Cauliflower Steak with Turmeric and Cumin

### Ingredients

- 1 large head cauliflower
- 2 tablespoons olive oil
- 1 teaspoon ground turmeric
- 1 teaspoon ground cumin
- 1/4 teaspoon ground black pepper
- 1 tablespoon fresh parsley, chopped

### Instructions

1. Preheat the oven to 400°F (200°C).
2. Remove the outer leaves of the cauliflower and trim the stem. Cut the cauliflower into 1-inch thick steaks.
3. In a small bowl, mix together olive oil, ground turmeric, ground cumin, and ground black pepper.
4. Brush the cauliflower steaks with the olive oil mixture, ensuring they are well coated.
5. Place the cauliflower steaks on a baking sheet lined with parchment paper.
6. Roast in the preheated oven for 25-30 minutes, flipping halfway through, until the cauliflower is tender and golden brown.
7. Remove from the oven and sprinkle with fresh parsley.
8. Serve warm.

### Nutrition Info per Serving

- Calories: 100
- Protein: 3g
- Carbohydrates: 8g
- Fiber: 3g
- Sugars: 2g
- Fat: 7g
- Saturated Fat: 1g
- Sodium: 45mg

**Servings: 4**
**Cooking Time: 35 minutes**

## 7. Eggplant Parmesan with Marinara Sauce

**Ingredients**

- 1 large eggplant, sliced into 1/2-inch rounds
- 2 tablespoons olive oil
- 2 cups marinara sauce (low sodium)
- 1 cup shredded mozzarella cheese (low-fat)
- 1/4 cup grated Parmesan cheese
- 1 teaspoon dried oregano
- 1/4 teaspoon ground black pepper
- 1/4 cup fresh basil, chopped

**Instructions**

1. Preheat the oven to 375°F (190°C).
2. Brush the eggplant slices with olive oil and place them on a baking sheet lined with parchment paper.
3. Bake in the preheated oven for 15-20 minutes, until the eggplant is tender.
4. In a baking dish, spread a thin layer of marinara sauce. Arrange a layer of eggplant slices on top of the sauce.
5. Sprinkle with a mixture of mozzarella and Parmesan cheese, then add a sprinkle of dried oregano and ground black pepper.
6. Repeat the layers until all the ingredients are used, finishing with a layer of cheese on top.
7. Bake in the preheated oven for 20-25 minutes, until the cheese is melted and bubbly.
8. Remove from the oven and let rest for a few minutes before serving.
9. Garnish with fresh basil.
10. Serve warm.

**Nutrition Info per Serving**

- Calories: 220
- Protein: 10g
- Carbohydrates: 18g
- Fiber: 6g
- Sugars: 8g
- Fat: 13g
- Saturated Fat: 4g
- Sodium: 320mg

**Servings: 4**
**Cooking Time: 45 minutes**

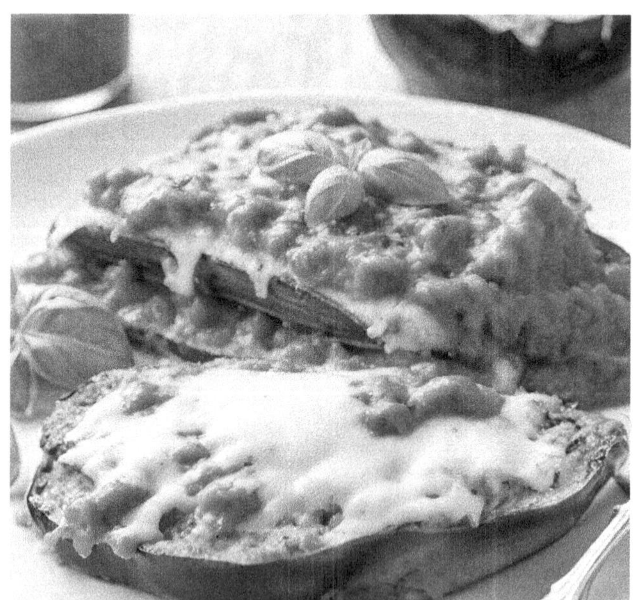

## 8. Spinach and Mushroom Frittata

### Ingredients

- 6 large eggs
- 1/4 cup unsweetened almond milk
- 1 tablespoon olive oil
- 1 small onion, diced
- 2 garlic cloves, minced
- 1 cup mushrooms, sliced
- 2 cups fresh spinach, chopped
- 1/4 teaspoon ground black pepper
- 1/4 cup grated Parmesan cheese

### Instructions

1. Preheat the oven to 350°F (175°C).
2. In a large bowl, whisk together the eggs and almond milk until well combined.
3. Heat olive oil in a large oven-safe skillet over medium heat.
4. Add diced onion and minced garlic to the skillet. Sauté for 3-4 minutes until the onion is translucent.
5. Add sliced mushrooms and cook for another 5 minutes until tender.
6. Add chopped spinach and cook for 2-3 minutes until wilted.
7. Pour the egg mixture into the skillet and stir gently to combine with the vegetables.
8. Sprinkle grated Parmesan cheese and ground black pepper over the top.
9. Transfer the skillet to the preheated oven and bake for 15-20 minutes, or until the frittata is set and the top is golden brown.
10. Remove from the oven and let cool slightly before slicing.
11. Serve warm.

### Nutrition Info per Serving

- Calories: 180
- Protein: 12g
- Carbohydrates: 5g
- Fiber: 2g
- Sugars: 2g
- Fat: 13g
- Saturated Fat: 3g
- Sodium: 180mg

Servings: 4

Cooking Time: 30 minutes

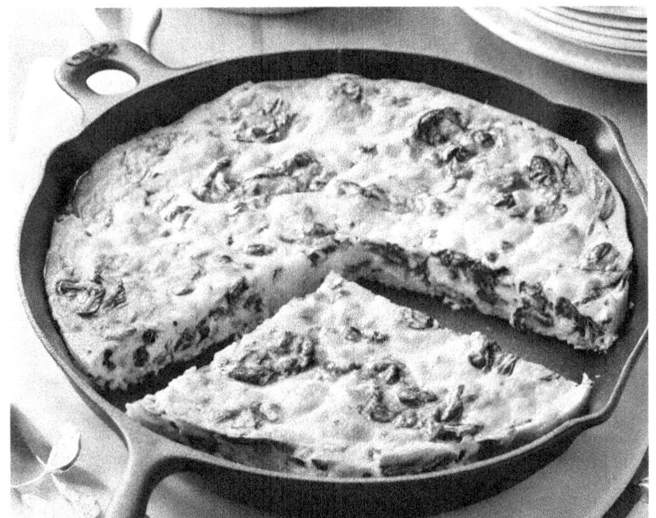

**9. Broccoli and Garlic Sauté**

**Ingredients**

- 4 cups broccoli florets
- 2 tablespoons olive oil
- 4 garlic cloves, thinly sliced
- 1/4 teaspoon ground black pepper
- 1 tablespoon lemon juice

**Instructions**

1. Heat olive oil in a large skillet over medium heat.
2. Add thinly sliced garlic to the skillet and sauté for 1-2 minutes until fragrant and lightly golden.
3. Add broccoli florets to the skillet and cook for 5-7 minutes, stirring occasionally, until the broccoli is tender but still crisp.
4. Sprinkle ground black pepper and lemon juice over the broccoli.
5. Cook for an additional 1-2 minutes until the broccoli is well coated.
6. Remove from heat and serve warm.

**Nutrition Info per Serving**

- Calories: 120
- Protein: 3g
- Carbohydrates: 10g
- Fiber: 4g
- Sugars: 2g
- Fat: 9g
- Saturated Fat: 1.5g
- Sodium: 35mg

**Servings: 4**
**Cooking Time: 15 minutes**

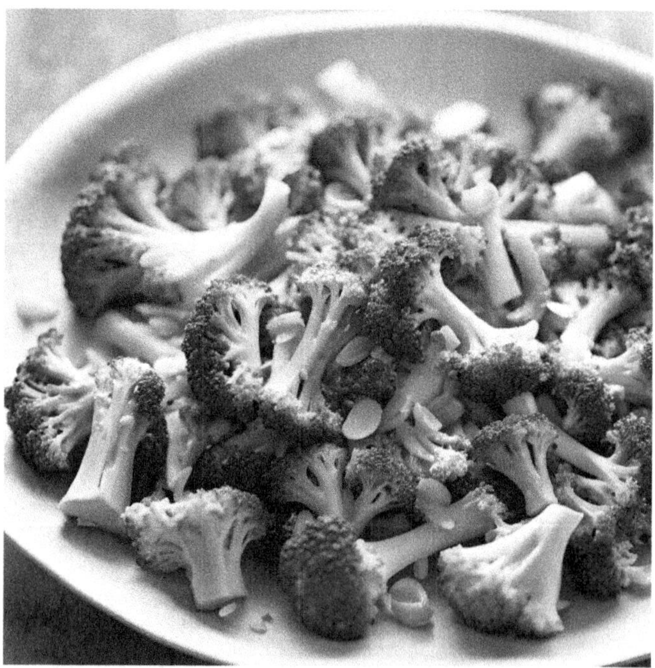

## 10. Stir-Fried Green Beans with Ginger

**Ingredients**

- 1 pound green beans, trimmed
- 1 tablespoon olive oil
- 1 tablespoon fresh ginger, grated
- 2 garlic cloves, minced
- 1 tablespoon low-sodium soy sauce
- 1 tablespoon sesame seeds
- 1/4 teaspoon ground black pepper

**Instructions**

1. Heat olive oil in a large skillet or wok over medium-high heat.
2. Add grated ginger and minced garlic to the skillet. Sauté for 1-2 minutes until fragrant.
3. Add green beans to the skillet and stir-fry for 5-7 minutes until tender but still crisp.
4. Stir in low-sodium soy sauce and ground black pepper. Cook for an additional 1-2 minutes until the green beans are well coated.
5. Sprinkle sesame seeds over the green beans and stir to combine.
6. Remove from heat and serve warm.

**Nutrition Info per Serving**

- Calories: 100
- Protein: 3g
- Carbohydrates: 8g
- Fiber: 3g
- Sugars: 2g
- Fat: 7g
- Saturated Fat: 1g
- Sodium: 140mg

**Servings: 4**
**Cooking Time: 15 minutes**

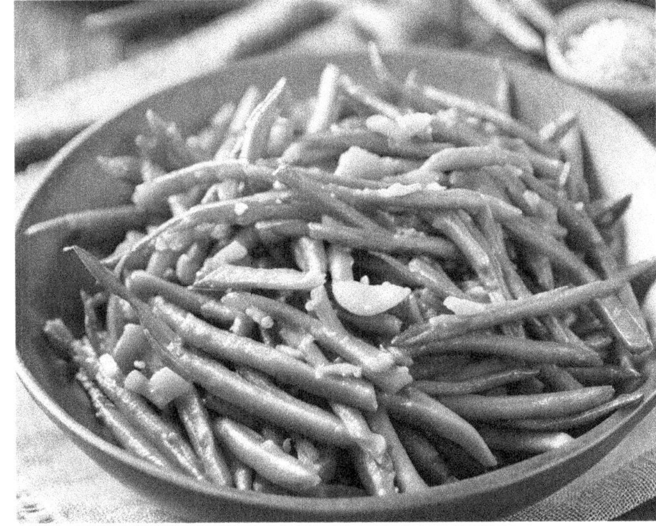

## 11. Ratatouille with Eggplant, Zucchini, and Bell Pepper

**Ingredients**

- 1 large eggplant, diced
- 2 zucchinis, diced
- 1 red bell pepper, diced
- 1 yellow bell pepper, diced
- 1 onion, diced
- 3 garlic cloves, minced
- 4 tomatoes, diced
- 1/4 cup olive oil
- 1 teaspoon dried thyme
- 1 teaspoon dried oregano
- 1/4 teaspoon ground black pepper
- 1/4 cup fresh basil, chopped

**Instructions**

1. Heat olive oil in a large pot over medium heat.
2. Add diced onion and minced garlic. Sauté for 3-4 minutes until the onion is translucent.
3. Add diced eggplant, zucchinis, red bell pepper, and yellow bell pepper. Cook for about 10 minutes, stirring occasionally, until the vegetables are tender.
4. Add diced tomatoes, dried thyme, dried oregano, and ground black pepper. Stir to combine.
5. Cover and simmer for 20-25 minutes, stirring occasionally, until all the vegetables are soft and the flavors are well blended.
6. Remove from heat and stir in fresh basil.
7. Serve warm.

**Nutrition Info per Serving**

- Calories: 150
- Protein: 2g
- Carbohydrates: 15g
- Fiber: 6g
- Sugars: 10g
- Fat: 10g
- Saturated Fat: 1.5g
- Sodium: 30mg

**Servings: 4**
**Cooking Time: 40 minutes**

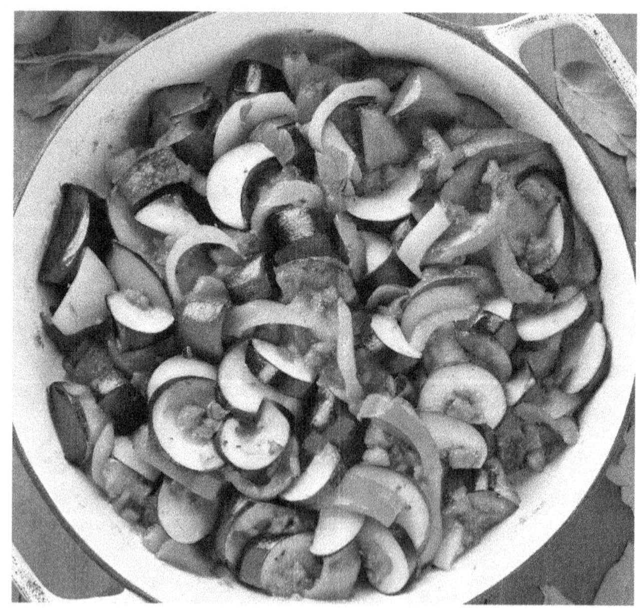

## 12. Spaghetti Squash with Tomato Sauce

### Ingredients

- 1 large spaghetti squash
- 2 tablespoons olive oil
- 1 onion, diced
- 3 garlic cloves, minced
- 4 tomatoes, diced
- 1 teaspoon dried basil
- 1 teaspoon dried oregano
- 1/4 teaspoon ground black pepper
- 1/4 cup grated Parmesan cheese (optional)
- 1/4 cup fresh parsley, chopped

### Instructions

1. Preheat the oven to 375°F (190°C).
2. Cut the spaghetti squash in half lengthwise and scoop out the seeds. Drizzle with 1 tablespoon of olive oil.
3. Place the squash halves cut-side down on a baking sheet and bake for 40-45 minutes, or until the flesh is tender.
4. While the squash is baking, heat the remaining olive oil in a large skillet over medium heat.
5. Add diced onion and minced garlic. Sauté for 3-4 minutes until the onion is translucent.
6. Add diced tomatoes, dried basil, dried oregano, and ground black pepper. Simmer for 20 minutes until the sauce thickens.
7. Remove the squash from the oven and use a fork to scrape the flesh into strands.
8. Serve the spaghetti squash topped with tomato sauce, grated Parmesan cheese (if using), and fresh parsley.

### Nutrition Info per Serving

- Calories: 180
- Protein: 4g
- Carbohydrates: 20g
- Fiber: 5g
- Sugars: 10g
- Fat: 10g
- Saturated Fat: 2g
- Sodium: 40mg

**Servings: 4**

**Cooking Time: 50 minutes**

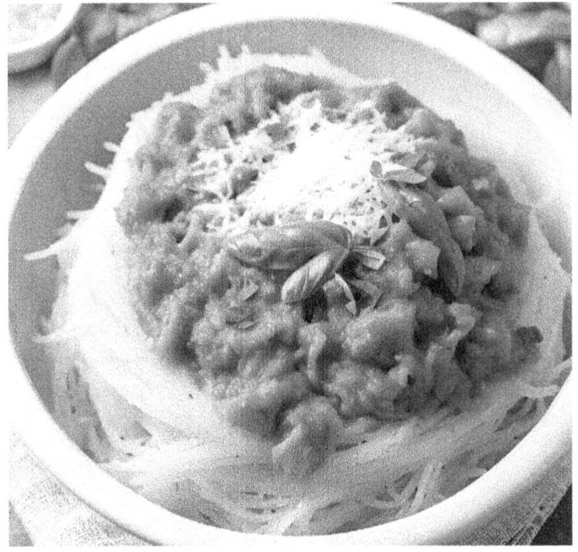

## 13. Avocado and Tomato Salad

**Ingredients**

- 2 ripe avocados, diced
- 1 cup cherry tomatoes, halved
- 1/4 cup red onion, finely chopped
- 2 tablespoons fresh cilantro, chopped
- 2 tablespoons olive oil
- 1 tablespoon lime juice
- 1/4 teaspoon ground black pepper

**Instructions**

1. In a large bowl, combine diced avocados, cherry tomatoes, red onion, and fresh cilantro.
2. In a small bowl, whisk together olive oil, lime juice, and ground black pepper.
3. Pour the dressing over the avocado and tomato mixture and toss gently to combine.
4. Serve immediately.

**Nutrition Info per Serving**

- Calories: 220
- Protein: 2g
- Carbohydrates: 10g
- Fiber: 6g
- Sugars: 2g
- Fat: 20g
- Saturated Fat: 3g
- Sodium: 10mg

**Servings: 4**
**Cooking Time: 10 minutes**

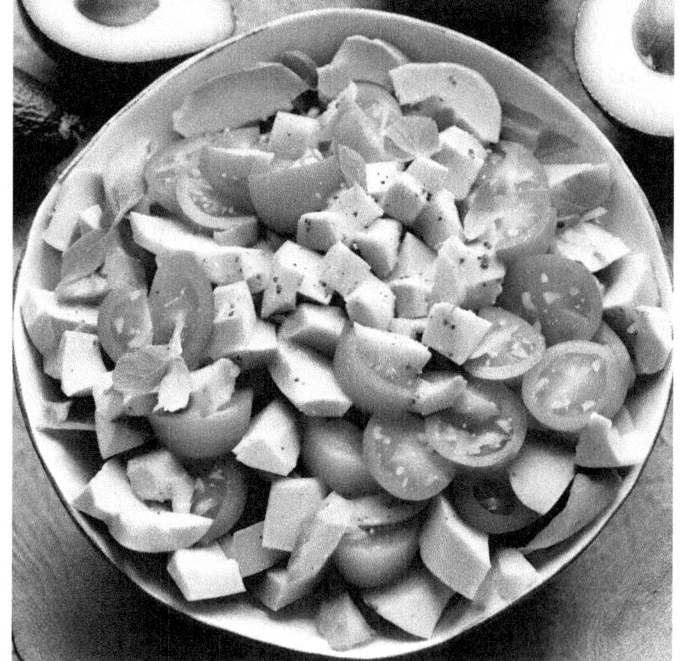

## 14. Creamy Pumpkin Risotto

**Ingredients**

- 1 cup Arborio rice
- 2 tablespoons olive oil
- 1 onion, finely chopped
- 2 garlic cloves, minced
- 1 cup pumpkin puree
- 4 cups low-sodium vegetable broth
- 1/4 cup unsweetened almond milk
- 1/4 teaspoon ground nutmeg
- 1/4 teaspoon ground black pepper
- 1/4 cup grated Parmesan cheese (optional)
- 1 tablespoon fresh sage, chopped

**Instructions**

1. In a medium pot, bring the vegetable broth to a simmer and keep warm.
2. In a large pot, heat olive oil over medium heat. Add finely chopped onion and minced garlic. Sauté for 3-4 minutes until the onion is translucent.
3. Add Arborio rice and cook, stirring constantly, for 2-3 minutes until the rice is lightly toasted.
4. Add the pumpkin puree and stir to combine.
5. Begin adding the warm vegetable broth one ladle at a time, stirring frequently, allowing the liquid to be absorbed before adding more. Continue this process until the rice is creamy and cooked through, about 18-20 minutes.
6. Stir in unsweetened almond milk, ground nutmeg, ground black pepper, and grated Parmesan cheese (if using).
7. Remove from heat and stir in fresh sage.
8. Serve warm.

**Nutrition Info per Serving**

- Calories: 250
- Protein: 5g
- Carbohydrates: 40g
- Fiber: 4g
- Sugars: 4g
- Fat: 8g
- Saturated Fat: 1.5g
- Sodium: 120mg

**Servings: 4**
**Cooking Time: 30 minutes**

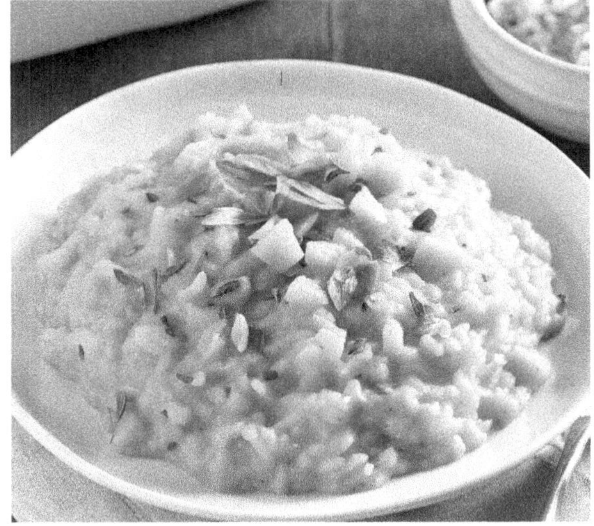

## 15. Sautéed Swiss Chard with Pine Nuts

**Ingredients**

- 1 bunch Swiss chard, stems removed and leaves chopped
- 2 tablespoons olive oil
- 3 garlic cloves, minced
- 1/4 cup pine nuts
- 1 tablespoon lemon juice
- 1/4 teaspoon ground black pepper

**Instructions**

1. Heat olive oil in a large skillet over medium heat.
2. Add minced garlic and sauté for 1-2 minutes until fragrant.
3. Add chopped Swiss chard and cook for 5-7 minutes until wilted and tender.
4. Stir in pine nuts and cook for an additional 2-3 minutes until the pine nuts are lightly toasted.
5. Remove from heat and stir in lemon juice and ground black pepper.
6. Serve warm.

**Nutrition Info per Serving**

- Calories: 160
- Protein: 3g
- Carbohydrates: 8g
- Fiber: 3g
- Sugars: 1g
- Fat: 14g
- Saturated Fat: 2g
- Sodium: 30mg

**Servings: 4**
**Cooking Time: 15 minutes**

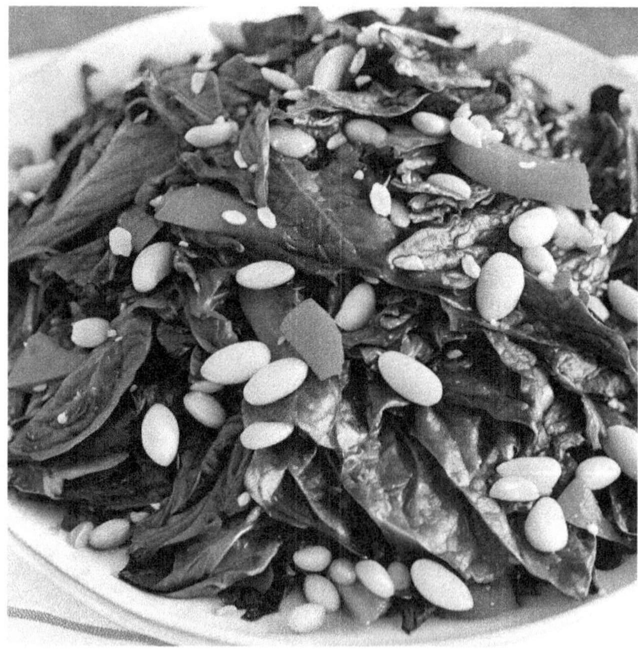

## 16. Curried Lentils with Carrots and Peas

### Ingredients

- 1 cup dried lentils, rinsed
- 2 tablespoons olive oil
- 1 onion, diced
- 2 garlic cloves, minced
- 2 carrots, diced
- 1 cup frozen peas
- 2 tablespoons curry powder
- 4 cups low-sodium vegetable broth
- 1/4 teaspoon ground cumin
- 1/4 teaspoon ground turmeric
- 1/4 teaspoon ground black pepper
- 1 tablespoon fresh cilantro, chopped

### Instructions

1. Heat olive oil in a large pot over medium heat.
2. Add diced onion and minced garlic. Sauté for 3-4 minutes until the onion is translucent.
3. Add diced carrots and cook for an additional 5 minutes.
4. Stir in curry powder, ground cumin, ground turmeric, and ground black pepper. Cook for 1 minute until fragrant.
5. Add lentils and vegetable broth. Bring to a boil, then reduce heat and simmer for 25-30 minutes until the lentils are tender.
6. Stir in frozen peas and cook for an additional 5 minutes until heated through.
7. Remove from heat and stir in fresh cilantro.
8. Serve warm.

### Nutrition Info per Serving

- Calories: 250
- Protein: 12g
- Carbohydrates: 40g
- Fiber: 15g
- Sugars: 7g
- Fat: 8g
- Saturated Fat: 1g
- Sodium: 200mg

**Servings: 4**
**Cooking Time: 40 minutes**

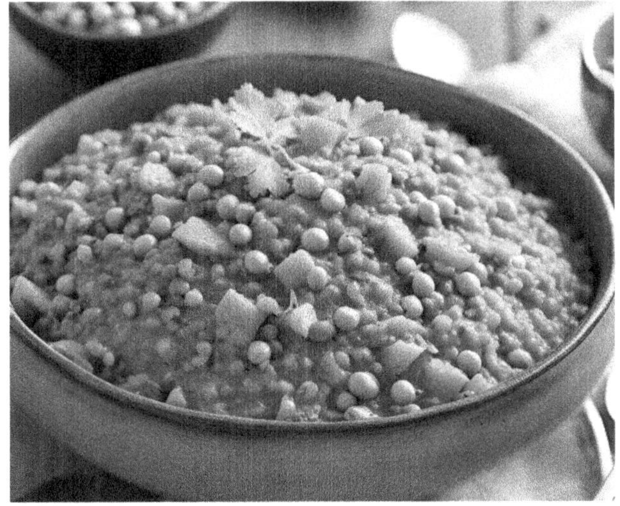

## 17. Vegetable Stuffed Portobello Mushrooms

**Ingredients**

- 4 large Portobello mushrooms, stems removed
- 2 tablespoons olive oil
- 1 small onion, diced
- 2 garlic cloves, minced
- 1 red bell pepper, diced
- 1 zucchini, diced
- 1/2 cup cherry tomatoes, halved
- 1/4 cup grated Parmesan cheese (optional)
- 1 teaspoon dried oregano
- 1/4 teaspoon ground black pepper
- 1 tablespoon fresh parsley, chopped

**Instructions**

1. Preheat the oven to 375°F (190°C).
2. Brush the Portobello mushrooms with 1 tablespoon of olive oil and place them on a baking sheet.
3. Bake in the preheated oven for 10 minutes.
4. While the mushrooms are baking, heat the remaining olive oil in a large skillet over medium heat.
5. Add diced onion and minced garlic. Sauté for 3-4 minutes until the onion is translucent.
6. Add diced red bell pepper and zucchini. Cook for 5-7 minutes until tender.
7. Stir in cherry tomatoes, dried oregano, and ground black pepper. Cook for an additional 2-3 minutes until the tomatoes are soft.
8. Remove the mushrooms from the oven and stuff them with the vegetable mixture.
9. Sprinkle with grated Parmesan cheese (if using).
10. Return the stuffed mushrooms to the oven and bake for an additional 10 minutes.
11. Remove from the oven and sprinkle with fresh parsley.
12. Serve warm.

**Nutrition Info per Serving**

- Calories: 180
- Protein: 5g
- Carbohydrates: 18g
- Fiber: 6g
- Sugars: 8g
- Fat: 10g
- Saturated Fat: 2g
- Sodium: 150mg

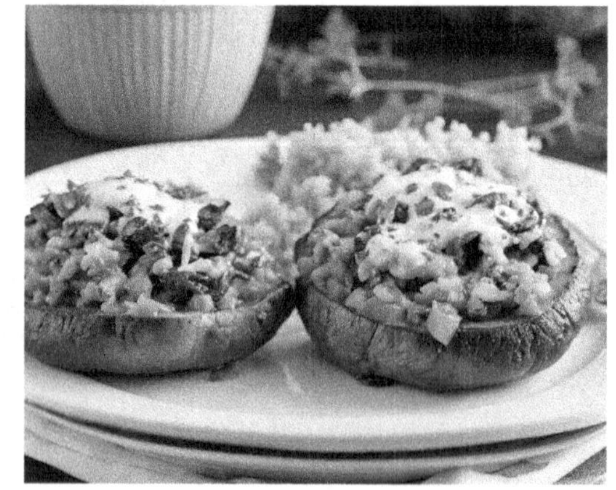

**Servings: 4**

**Cooking Time: 30 minutes**

## 18. Sweet Corn and Zucchini Pie

**Ingredients**

- 1 cup whole wheat flour
- 1/2 cup cornmeal
- 1 teaspoon baking powder
- 1/4 teaspoon ground black pepper
- 2 tablespoons olive oil
- 1/2 cup unsweetened almond milk
- 1 egg, beaten
- 1 cup fresh corn kernels
- 1 zucchini, grated
- 1/2 cup cherry tomatoes, halved
- 1/4 cup grated Parmesan cheese (optional)
- 1 tablespoon fresh basil, chopped

**Instructions**

1. Preheat the oven to 375°F (190°C).
2. In a large bowl, mix together whole wheat flour, cornmeal, baking powder, and ground black pepper.
3. In a separate bowl, whisk together olive oil, almond milk, and beaten egg.
4. Add the wet ingredients to the dry ingredients and mix until just combined.
5. Fold in fresh corn kernels, grated zucchini, cherry tomatoes, and grated Parmesan cheese (if using).
6. Pour the batter into a greased pie dish.
7. Bake in the preheated oven for 25-30 minutes, or until the top is golden brown and a toothpick inserted into the center comes out clean.
8. Remove from the oven and let cool for a few minutes.
9. Sprinkle with fresh basil.
10. Serve warm.

**Nutrition Info per Serving**

- Calories: 200
- Protein: 6g
- Carbohydrates: 26g
- Fiber: 4g
- Sugars: 3g
- Fat: 8g
- Saturated Fat: 1.5g
- Sodium: 150mg

**Servings: 4**
**Cooking Time: 40 minutes**

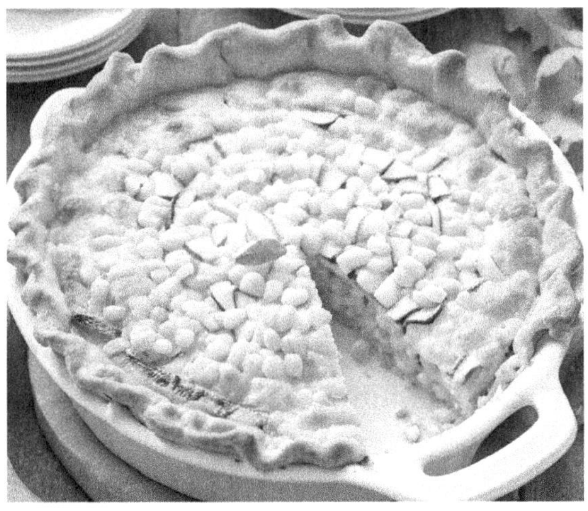

**19. Vegetarian Stew with Barley and Winter Squash**

**Ingredients**

- 1 cup pearl barley, rinsed
- 2 tablespoons olive oil
- 1 onion, diced
- 2 garlic cloves, minced
- 2 cups butternut squash, peeled and cubed
- 2 carrots, sliced
- 2 celery stalks, sliced
- 4 cups low-sodium vegetable broth
- 1 teaspoon dried thyme
- 1/4 teaspoon ground black pepper
- 1 cup kale, chopped

**Instructions**

1. Heat olive oil in a large pot over medium heat.
2. Add diced onion and minced garlic. Sauté for 3-4 minutes until the onion is translucent.
3. Add butternut squash, carrots, and celery. Cook for 5-7 minutes until the vegetables are slightly tender.
4. Stir in pearl barley, vegetable broth, dried thyme, and ground black pepper. Bring to a boil.
5. Reduce heat and simmer for 30-35 minutes, or until the barley is tender and the vegetables are cooked through.
6. Stir in chopped kale and cook for an additional 5 minutes until wilted.
7. Remove from heat and let cool slightly before serving.
8. Serve warm.

**Nutrition Info per Serving**

- Calories: 250
- Protein: 6g
- Carbohydrates: 45g
- Fiber: 10g
- Sugars: 8g
- Fat: 7g
- Saturated Fat: 1g
- Sodium: 220mg

**Servings: 4**

**Cooking Time: 45 minutes**

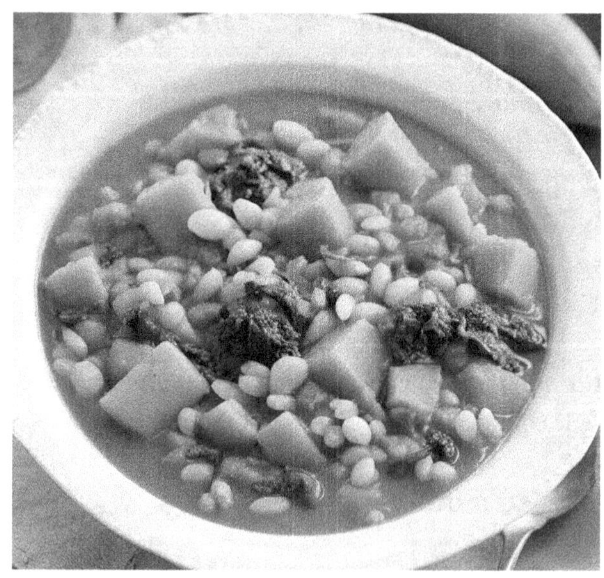

## 20. Warm Quinoa and Roasted Vegetable Salad

### Ingredients

- 1 cup quinoa, rinsed
- 2 cups low-sodium vegetable broth
- 2 tablespoons olive oil
- 1 red bell pepper, diced
- 1 zucchini, diced
- 1 cup cherry tomatoes, halved
- 1 small red onion, sliced
- 1 teaspoon dried oregano
- 1/4 teaspoon ground black pepper
- 1 tablespoon balsamic vinegar
- 1/4 cup fresh parsley, chopped

### Instructions

1. Preheat the oven to 400°F (200°C).
2. In a medium pot, bring the vegetable broth to a boil. Add quinoa, reduce heat to low, cover, and simmer for 15 minutes, or until the quinoa is cooked and the liquid is absorbed.
3. In a large bowl, combine diced red bell pepper, zucchini, cherry tomatoes, and sliced red onion. Toss with olive oil, dried oregano, and ground black pepper.
4. Spread the vegetables on a baking sheet lined with parchment paper.
5. Roast in the preheated oven for 20-25 minutes, or until the vegetables are tender and slightly caramelized.
6. In a large bowl, combine cooked quinoa and roasted vegetables. Drizzle with balsamic vinegar and toss to combine.
7. Sprinkle with fresh parsley.
8. Serve warm.

### Nutrition Info per Serving

- Calories: 230
- Protein: 6g
- Carbohydrates: 30g
- Fiber: 5g
- Sugars: 6g
- Fat: 10g
- Saturated Fat: 1.5g
- Sodium: 120mg

**Servings: 4**

**Cooking Time: 35 minutes**

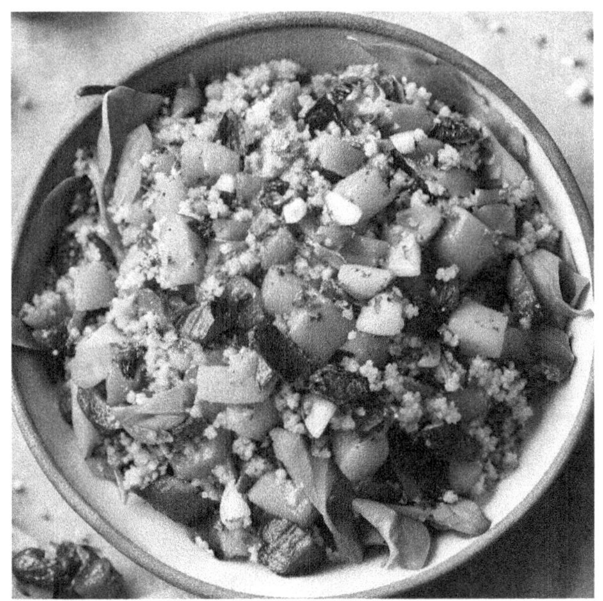

## 21. Roasted Turnips with Maple and Mustard

**Ingredients**

- 1 pound turnips, peeled and cubed
- 2 tablespoons olive oil
- 1 tablespoon maple syrup
- 1 tablespoon Dijon mustard
- 1/4 teaspoon ground black pepper
- 1 tablespoon fresh thyme, chopped

**Instructions**

1. Preheat the oven to 400°F (200°C).
2. In a large bowl, whisk together olive oil, maple syrup, Dijon mustard, and ground black pepper.
3. Add the cubed turnips to the bowl and toss to coat evenly.
4. Spread the turnips on a baking sheet lined with parchment paper.
5. Roast in the preheated oven for 25-30 minutes, or until the turnips are tender and golden brown, stirring halfway through.
6. Remove from the oven and sprinkle with fresh thyme.
7. Serve warm.

**Nutrition Info per Serving**

- Calories: 130
- Protein: 2g
- Carbohydrates: 15g
- Fiber: 3g
- Sugars: 7g
- Fat: 7g
- Saturated Fat: 1g
- Sodium: 120mg

**Servings: 4**

**Cooking Time: 30 minutes**

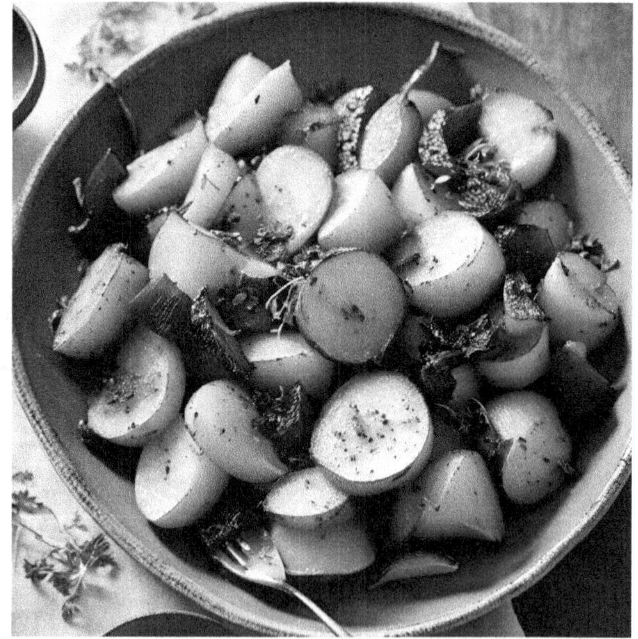

# Soup and Stew Recipes

**1. Hearty Turkey and Vegetable Stew**
**Ingredients**

- 1 pound ground turkey
- 2 tablespoons olive oil
- 1 onion, diced
- 2 garlic cloves, minced
- 3 carrots, sliced
- 2 celery stalks, sliced
- 2 potatoes, peeled and diced
- 1 cup green beans, trimmed and cut into 1-inch pieces
- 4 cups low-sodium chicken broth
- 1 teaspoon dried thyme
- 1/4 teaspoon ground black pepper
- 1 bay leaf
- 1 tablespoon fresh parsley, chopped

**Instructions**

1. Heat olive oil in a large pot over medium heat.
2. Add ground turkey and cook until browned, about 5-7 minutes.
3. Add diced onion and minced garlic. Sauté for 3-4 minutes until the onion is translucent.
4. Add sliced carrots, celery, and potatoes. Cook for 5-7 minutes until the vegetables are slightly tender.
5. Stir in green beans, chicken broth, dried thyme, ground black pepper, and bay leaf.
6. Bring to a boil, then reduce heat and simmer for 30-35 minutes until the vegetables are tender.
7. Remove the bay leaf and stir in fresh parsley.
8. Serve warm.

**Nutrition Info per Serving**

- Calories: 250
- Protein: 20g
- Carbohydrates: 25g
- Fiber: 5g
- Sugars: 6g
- Fat: 10g
- Saturated Fat: 2g
- Sodium: 200mg

**Servings: 4**
**Cooking Time: 45 minutes**

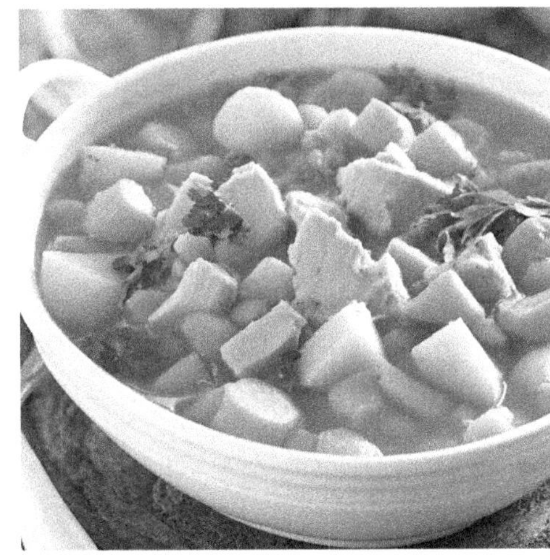

## 2. Lentil and Spinach Soup

**Ingredients**

- 1 cup dried lentils, rinsed
- 2 tablespoons olive oil
- 1 onion, diced
- 2 garlic cloves, minced
- 2 carrots, diced
- 2 celery stalks, diced
- 4 cups low-sodium vegetable broth
- 1 teaspoon ground cumin
- 1/4 teaspoon ground black pepper
- 4 cups fresh spinach, chopped
- 1 tablespoon fresh lemon juice

**Instructions**

1. Heat olive oil in a large pot over medium heat.
2. Add diced onion and minced garlic. Sauté for 3-4 minutes until the onion is translucent.
3. Add diced carrots and celery. Cook for 5-7 minutes until the vegetables are slightly tender.
4. Stir in lentils, vegetable broth, ground cumin, and ground black pepper. Bring to a boil.
5. Reduce heat and simmer for 25-30 minutes until the lentils are tender.
6. Stir in chopped spinach and cook for an additional 5 minutes until wilted.
7. Remove from heat and stir in fresh lemon juice.
8. Serve warm.

**Nutrition Info per Serving**

- Calories: 220
- Protein: 10g
- Carbohydrates: 28g
- Fiber: 10g
- Sugars: 6g
- Fat: 8g
- Saturated Fat: 1g
- Sodium: 180mg

**Servings: 4**
**Cooking Time: 40 minutes**

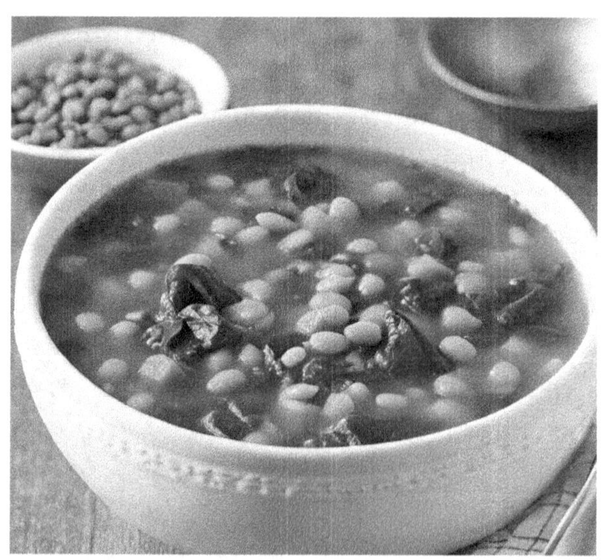

## 3. Fish Soup with Tomatoes and Herbs

### Ingredients

- 1 pound white fish fillets (such as cod or haddock), cut into chunks
- 2 tablespoons olive oil
- 1 onion, diced
- 2 garlic cloves, minced
- 4 tomatoes, diced
- 4 cups low-sodium fish or vegetable broth
- 1 teaspoon dried basil
- 1 teaspoon dried oregano
- 1/4 teaspoon ground black pepper
- 1 bay leaf
- 1 tablespoon fresh parsley, chopped

### Instructions

1. Heat olive oil in a large pot over medium heat.
2. Add diced onion and minced garlic. Sauté for 3-4 minutes until the onion is translucent.
3. Add diced tomatoes and cook for 5 minutes until they start to break down.
4. Stir in fish or vegetable broth, dried basil, dried oregano, ground black pepper, and bay leaf. Bring to a boil.
5. Reduce heat and simmer for 10 minutes.
6. Add fish chunks and cook for an additional 10 minutes until the fish is cooked through and opaque.
7. Remove the bay leaf and stir in fresh parsley.
8. Serve warm.

### Nutrition Info per Serving

- Calories: 200
- Protein: 25g
- Carbohydrates: 10g
- Fiber: 3g
- Sugars: 6g
- Fat: 8g
- Saturated Fat: 1.5g
- Sodium: 180mg

**Servings: 4**

**Cooking Time: 35 minutes**

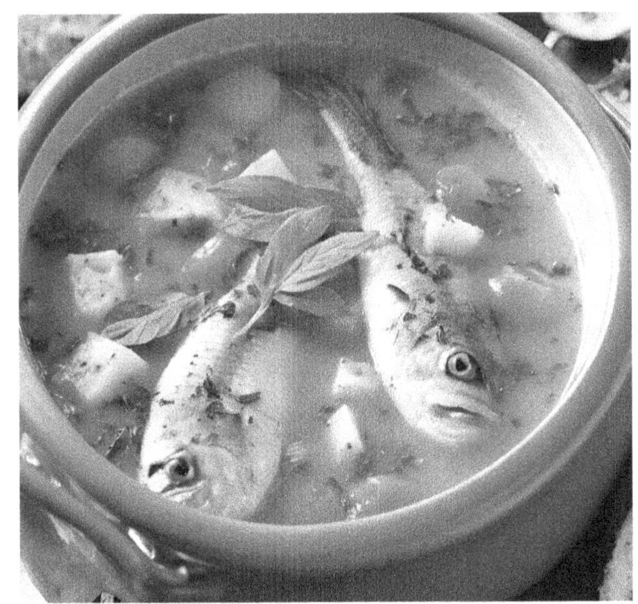

**4. White Bean and Escarole Soup**
**Ingredients**

- 2 tablespoons olive oil
- 1 onion, diced
- 2 garlic cloves, minced
- 1 head escarole, chopped
- 4 cups low-sodium vegetable broth
- 2 cans (15 ounces each) white beans, drained and rinsed
- 1 teaspoon dried thyme
- 1/4 teaspoon ground black pepper
- 1 tablespoon fresh lemon juice
- 1/4 cup grated Parmesan cheese (optional)

**Instructions**

1. Heat olive oil in a large pot over medium heat.
2. Add diced onion and minced garlic. Sauté for 3-4 minutes until the onion is translucent.
3. Add chopped escarole and cook for 5-7 minutes until wilted.
4. Stir in vegetable broth, white beans, dried thyme, and ground black pepper. Bring to a boil.
5. Reduce heat and simmer for 20 minutes until the flavors are well combined.
6. Remove from heat and stir in fresh lemon juice.
7. Serve warm, topped with grated Parmesan cheese if desired.

**Nutrition Info per Serving**

- Calories: 220
- Protein: 10g
- Carbohydrates: 28g
- Fiber: 8g
- Sugars: 3g
- Fat: 8g
- Saturated Fat: 1.5g
- Sodium: 180mg

**Servings: 4**
**Cooking Time: 30 minutes**

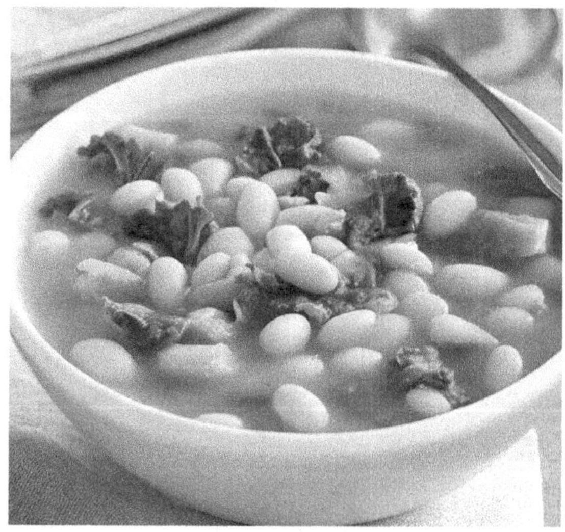

## 5. Vegetable Minestrone

**Ingredients**

- 2 tablespoons olive oil
- 1 onion, diced
- 2 garlic cloves, minced
- 2 carrots, diced
- 2 celery stalks, diced
- 1 zucchini, diced
- 1 cup green beans, trimmed and cut into 1-inch pieces
- 1 can (15 ounces) diced tomatoes
- 4 cups low-sodium vegetable broth
- 1 teaspoon dried basil
- 1 teaspoon dried oregano
- 1/4 teaspoon ground black pepper
- 1 can (15 ounces) kidney beans, drained and rinsed
- 1 cup small pasta (such as ditalini or elbow macaroni)
- 1/4 cup grated Parmesan cheese (optional)
- 1/4 cup fresh basil, chopped

**Instructions**

1. Heat olive oil in a large pot over medium heat.
2. Add diced onion and minced garlic. Sauté for 3-4 minutes until the onion is translucent.
3. Add diced carrots, celery, zucchini, and green beans. Cook for 5-7 minutes until the vegetables are slightly tender.
4. Stir in diced tomatoes, vegetable broth, dried basil, dried oregano, and ground black pepper. Bring to a boil.
5. Reduce heat and simmer for 15 minutes.
6. Add kidney beans and pasta. Cook for an additional 10-12 minutes until the pasta is al dente.
7. Remove from heat and stir in fresh basil.
8. Serve warm, topped with grated Parmesan cheese if desired.

**Nutrition Info per Serving**

- Calories: 280
- Protein: 10g
- Carbohydrates: 45g
- Fiber: 10g
- Sugars: 8g
- Fat: 8g
- Saturated Fat: 1.5g
- Sodium: 220mg

**Servings: 4**
**Cooking Time: 35 minutes**

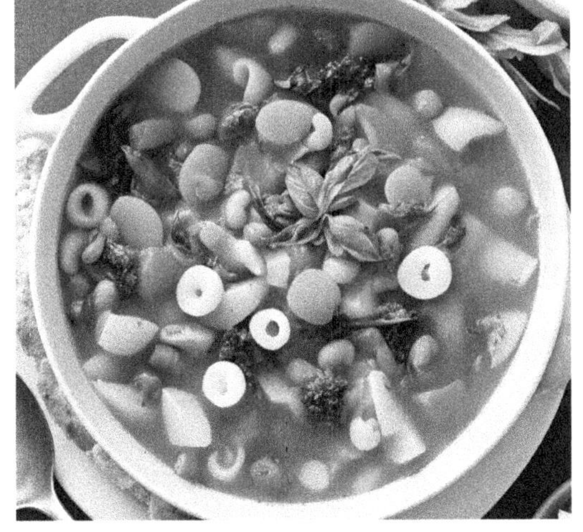

## 6. Chicken and Rice Soup with Lemon

### Ingredients

- 2 tablespoons olive oil
- 1 onion, diced
- 2 garlic cloves, minced
- 2 carrots, sliced
- 2 celery stalks, sliced
- 1 cup brown rice
- 6 cups low-sodium chicken broth
- 2 cups cooked chicken breast, shredded
- 1 teaspoon dried thyme
- 1/4 teaspoon ground black pepper
- 1 lemon, juiced and zested
- 1/4 cup fresh parsley, chopped

### Instructions

1. Heat olive oil in a large pot over medium heat.
2. Add diced onion and minced garlic. Sauté for 3-4 minutes until the onion is translucent.
3. Add sliced carrots and celery. Cook for 5-7 minutes until the vegetables are slightly tender.
4. Stir in brown rice, chicken broth, dried thyme, and ground black pepper. Bring to a boil.
5. Reduce heat and simmer for 30-35 minutes until the rice is cooked.
6. Add shredded chicken, lemon juice, and lemon zest. Cook for an additional 5 minutes.
7. Remove from heat and stir in fresh parsley.
8. Serve warm.

### Nutrition Info per Serving

- Calories: 250
- Protein: 18g
- Carbohydrates: 30g
- Fiber: 4g
- Sugars: 4g
- Fat: 8g
- Saturated Fat: 1.5g
- Sodium: 200mg

**Servings: 4**
**Cooking Time: 45 minutes**

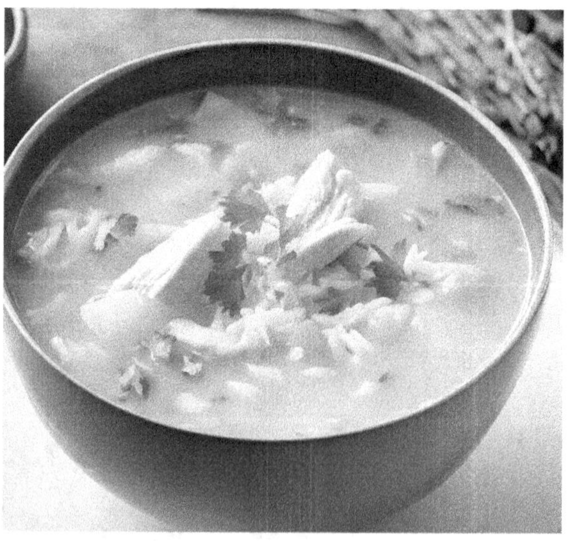

# 7. Miso Soup with Tofu and Seaweed

## Ingredients

- 4 cups water
- 1/4 cup miso paste
- 1 cup tofu, cubed
- 1/4 cup dried seaweed (wakame), soaked and drained
- 1 green onion, sliced
- 1 tablespoon low-sodium soy sauce
- 1/4 teaspoon ground black pepper

## Instructions

1. In a medium pot, bring water to a simmer over medium heat.
2. Add miso paste and whisk until fully dissolved.
3. Stir in cubed tofu, soaked seaweed, and soy sauce. Simmer for 5 minutes until the tofu is heated through.
4. Add sliced green onion and ground black pepper. Cook for an additional 1-2 minutes.
5. Remove from heat and serve warm.

## Nutrition Info per Serving

- Calories: 90
- Protein: 6g
- Carbohydrates: 8g
- Fiber: 2g
- Sugars: 1g
- Fat: 4g
- Saturated Fat: 0.5g
- Sodium: 300mg

**Servings: 4**
**Cooking Time: 15 minutes**

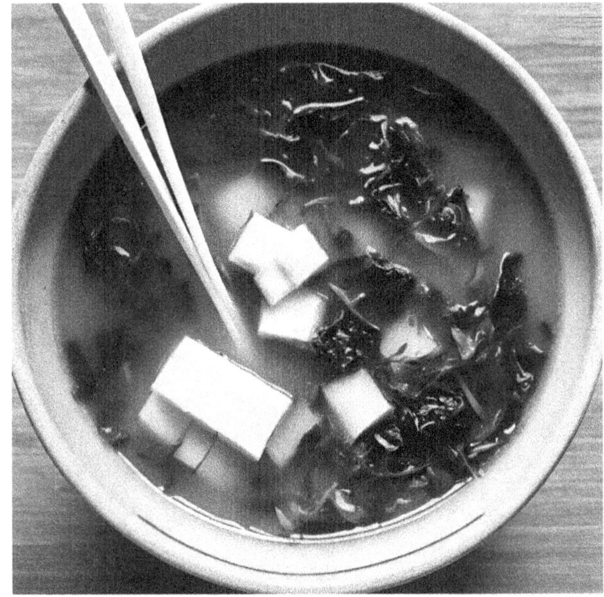

## 8. Beef Stew with Root Vegetables

**Ingredients**

- 1 pound beef stew meat, cubed
- 2 tablespoons olive oil
- 1 onion, diced
- 2 garlic cloves, minced
- 3 carrots, diced
- 2 parsnips, diced
- 2 potatoes, diced
- 4 cups low-sodium beef broth
- 1 teaspoon dried thyme
- 1 teaspoon dried rosemary
- 1/4 teaspoon ground black pepper
- 1 bay leaf

**Instructions**

1. Heat olive oil in a large pot over medium heat.
2. Add cubed beef stew meat and brown on all sides, about 5-7 minutes.
3. Add diced onion and minced garlic. Sauté for 3-4 minutes until the onion is translucent.
4. Stir in diced carrots, parsnips, and potatoes. Cook for 5-7 minutes until the vegetables are slightly tender.
5. Add beef broth, dried thyme, dried rosemary, ground black pepper, and bay leaf. Bring to a boil.
6. Reduce heat and simmer for 45-50 minutes until the beef and vegetables are tender.
7. Remove the bay leaf before serving.
8. Serve warm.

**Nutrition Info per Serving**

- Calories: 300
- Protein: 25g
- Carbohydrates: 20g
- Fiber: 4g
- Sugars: 5g
- Fat: 12g
- Saturated Fat: 3.5g
- Sodium: 250mg

**Servings: 4**
**Cooking Time: 60 minutes**

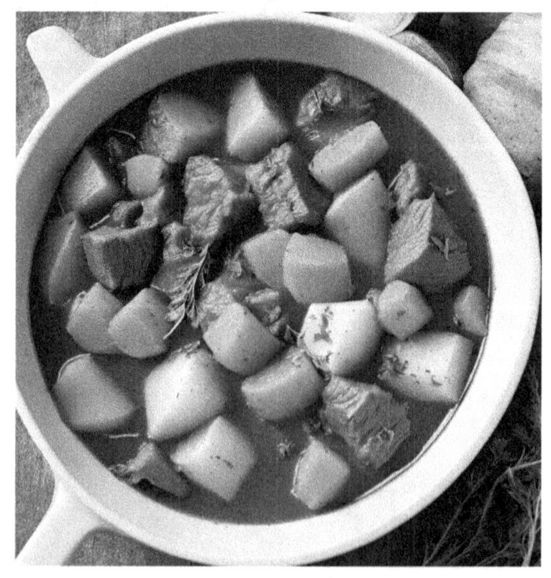

## 9. Barley and Mushroom Stew

**Ingredients**

- 2 tablespoons olive oil
- 1 onion, diced
- 2 garlic cloves, minced
- 2 cups mushrooms, sliced
- 1 cup pearl barley, rinsed
- 4 cups low-sodium vegetable broth
- 1 teaspoon dried thyme
- 1/4 teaspoon ground black pepper
- 2 carrots, diced
- 2 celery stalks, diced
- 1 bay leaf
- 1 tablespoon fresh parsley, chopped

**Instructions**

1. Heat olive oil in a large pot over medium heat.
2. Add diced onion and minced garlic. Sauté for 3-4 minutes until the onion is translucent.
3. Add sliced mushrooms and cook for 5 minutes until tender.
4. Stir in rinsed pearl barley, vegetable broth, dried thyme, ground black pepper, diced carrots, diced celery, and bay leaf. Bring to a boil.
5. Reduce heat and simmer for 40-45 minutes until the barley and vegetables are tender.
6. Remove the bay leaf and stir in fresh parsley.
7. Serve warm.

**Nutrition Info per Serving**

- Calories: 220
- Protein: 7g
- Carbohydrates: 35g
- Fiber: 8g
- Sugars: 7g
- Fat: 8g
- Saturated Fat: 1g
- Sodium: 180mg

**Servings: 4**
**Cooking Time: 50 minutes**

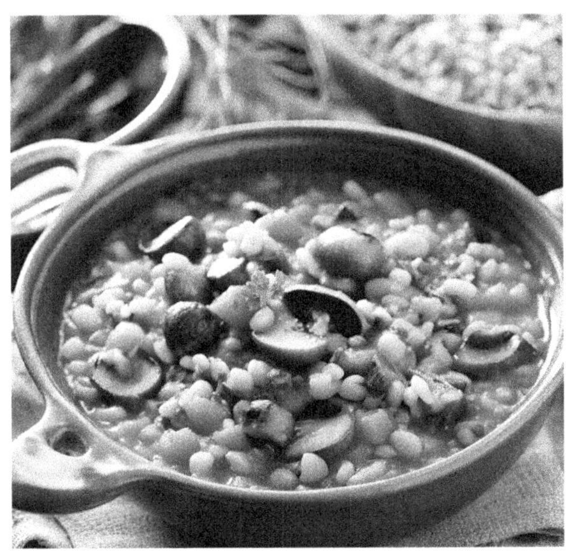

## 10. Shrimp and Corn Chowder

**Ingredients**

- 2 tablespoons olive oil
- 1 onion, diced
- 2 garlic cloves, minced
- 2 cups corn kernels (fresh or frozen)
- 1 pound shrimp, peeled and deveined
- 4 cups low-sodium chicken broth
- 1 cup unsweetened almond milk
- 1 teaspoon dried thyme
- 1/4 teaspoon ground black pepper
- 2 potatoes, diced
- 1 tablespoon fresh parsley, chopped

**Instructions**

1. Heat olive oil in a large pot over medium heat.
2. Add diced onion and minced garlic. Sauté for 3-4 minutes until the onion is translucent.
3. Stir in corn kernels and diced potatoes. Cook for 5-7 minutes until the vegetables are slightly tender.
4. Add chicken broth, unsweetened almond milk, dried thyme, and ground black pepper. Bring to a boil.
5. Reduce heat and simmer for 20 minutes until the potatoes are tender.
6. Add shrimp and cook for an additional 5 minutes until the shrimp are pink and opaque.
7. Remove from heat and stir in fresh parsley.
8. Serve warm.

**Nutrition Info per Serving**

- Calories: 250
- Protein: 18g
- Carbohydrates: 28g
- Fiber: 4g
- Sugars: 5g
- Fat: 8g
- Saturated Fat: 1g
- Sodium: 220mg

**Servings: 4**
**Cooking Time: 35 minutes**

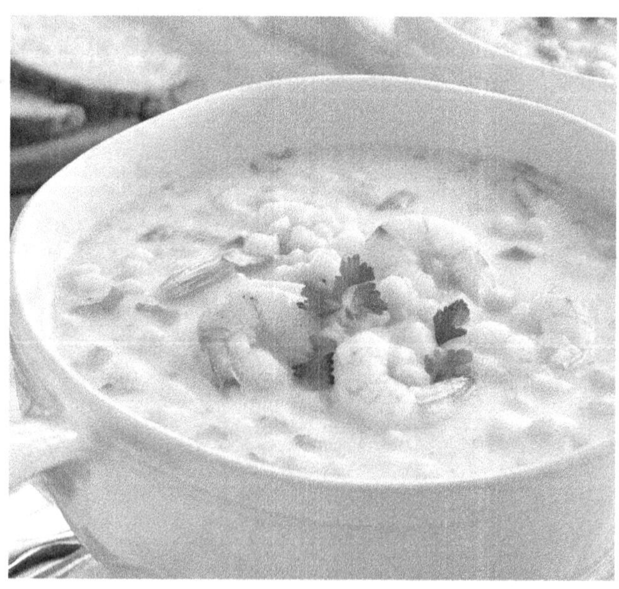

## 11. Moroccan Vegetable Stew with Chickpeas

**Ingredients**

- 2 tablespoons olive oil
- 1 onion, diced
- 3 garlic cloves, minced
- 2 carrots, sliced
- 2 zucchinis, diced
- 1 red bell pepper, diced
- 1 can (15 ounces) chickpeas, drained and rinsed
- 1 can (15 ounces) diced tomatoes
- 4 cups low-sodium vegetable broth
- 1 teaspoon ground cumin
- 1 teaspoon ground coriander
- 1 teaspoon ground cinnamon
- 1/4 teaspoon ground black pepper
- 1/2 cup dried apricots, chopped
- 1/4 cup fresh cilantro, chopped

**Instructions**

1. Heat olive oil in a large pot over medium heat.
2. Add diced onion and minced garlic. Sauté for 3-4 minutes until the onion is translucent.
3. Add sliced carrots, diced zucchinis, and red bell pepper. Cook for 5-7 minutes until the vegetables are slightly tender.
4. Stir in chickpeas, diced tomatoes, vegetable broth, ground cumin, ground coriander, ground cinnamon, and ground black pepper. Bring to a boil.
5. Reduce heat and simmer for 25-30 minutes until the vegetables are tender.
6. Stir in chopped apricots and cook for an additional 5 minutes.
7. Remove from heat and stir in fresh cilantro.
8. Serve warm.

**Nutrition Info per Serving**

- Calories: 300
- Protein: 8g
- Carbohydrates: 45g
- Fiber: 10g
- Sugars: 20g
- Fat: 10g
- Saturated Fat: 1.5g
- Sodium: 200mg

**Servings: 4**
**Cooking Time: 45 minutes**

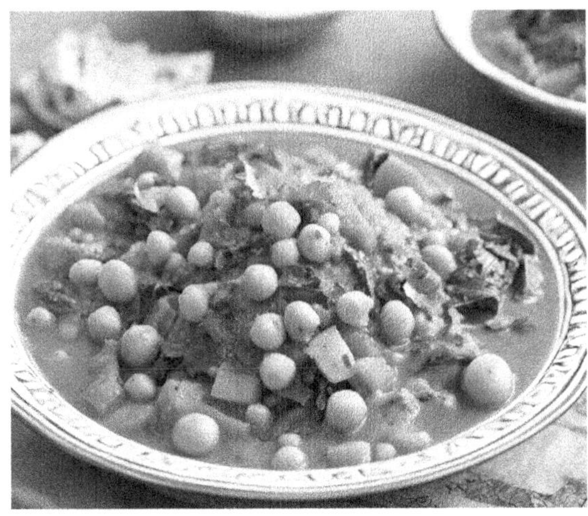

## 12. Vegan Mushroom and Tarragon Soup

**Ingredients**

- 2 tablespoons olive oil
- 1 onion, diced
- 3 garlic cloves, minced
- 4 cups mushrooms, sliced
- 4 cups low-sodium vegetable broth
- 1 cup unsweetened almond milk
- 1 teaspoon dried tarragon
- 1/4 teaspoon ground black pepper
- 2 tablespoons nutritional yeast
- 1 tablespoon fresh parsley, chopped

**Instructions**

1. Heat olive oil in a large pot over medium heat.
2. Add diced onion and minced garlic. Sauté for 3-4 minutes until the onion is translucent.
3. Add sliced mushrooms and cook for 5-7 minutes until tender.
4. Stir in vegetable broth, almond milk, dried tarragon, ground black pepper, and nutritional yeast. Bring to a boil.
5. Reduce heat and simmer for 20 minutes.
6. Remove from heat and stir in fresh parsley.
7. Serve warm.

**Nutrition Info per Serving**

- Calories: 150
- Protein: 5g
- Carbohydrates: 10g
- Fiber: 3g
- Sugars: 4g
- Fat: 10g
- Saturated Fat: 1.5g
- Sodium: 180mg

**Servings: 4**
**Cooking Time: 30 minutes**

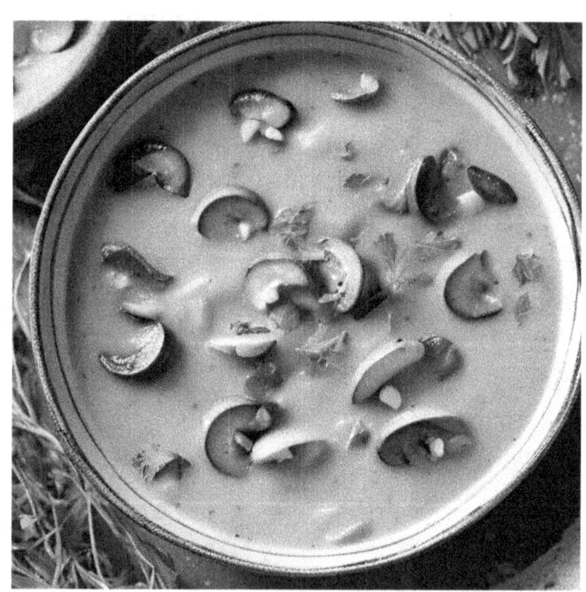

## 13. Italian Wedding Soup with Turkey Meatballs

**Ingredients**

- 1 pound ground turkey
- 1/4 cup whole wheat breadcrumbs
- 1 egg, beaten
- 2 tablespoons fresh parsley, chopped
- 1/4 teaspoon ground black pepper
- 2 tablespoons olive oil
- 1 onion, diced
- 2 garlic cloves, minced
- 2 carrots, diced
- 2 celery stalks, diced
- 4 cups low-sodium chicken broth
- 1 cup small pasta (such as acini di pepe)
- 4 cups fresh spinach, chopped

**Instructions**

1. In a large bowl, combine ground turkey, whole wheat breadcrumbs, beaten egg, fresh parsley, and ground black pepper. Mix well and form into small meatballs.
2. Heat olive oil in a large pot over medium heat. Add the meatballs and cook until browned on all sides, about 5-7 minutes. Remove meatballs from the pot and set aside.
3. In the same pot, add diced onion and minced garlic. Sauté for 3-4 minutes until the onion is translucent.
4. Add diced carrots and celery. Cook for 5-7 minutes until the vegetables are slightly tender.
5. Stir in chicken broth and bring to a boil.
6. Add the browned meatballs and pasta. Reduce heat and simmer for 10-12 minutes until the pasta is al dente.
7. Stir in chopped spinach and cook for an additional 2-3 minutes until wilted.
8. Serve warm.

**Nutrition Info per Serving**

- Calories: 300
- Protein: 25g
- Carbohydrates: 25g
- Fiber: 4g
- Sugars: 5g
- Fat: 12g
- Saturated Fat: 2.5g
- Sodium: 250mg

**Servings: 4**
**Cooking Time: 40 minutes**

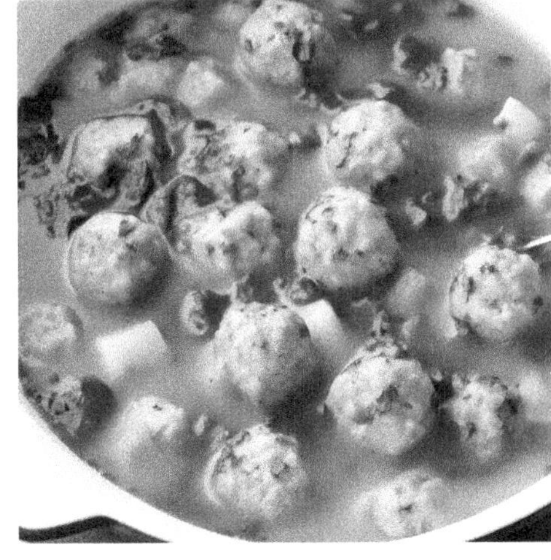

## 14. Pumpkin and Coconut Milk Soup

**Ingredients**

- 2 tablespoons olive oil
- 1 onion, diced
- 3 garlic cloves, minced
- 4 cups pumpkin puree
- 4 cups low-sodium vegetable broth
- 1 can (13.5 ounces) coconut milk
- 1 teaspoon ground ginger
- 1/4 teaspoon ground black pepper
- 1 tablespoon fresh cilantro, chopped

**Instructions**

1. Heat olive oil in a large pot over medium heat.
2. Add diced onion and minced garlic. Sauté for 3-4 minutes until the onion is translucent.
3. Stir in pumpkin puree, vegetable broth, coconut milk, ground ginger, and ground black pepper. Bring to a boil.
4. Reduce heat and simmer for 20 minutes, stirring occasionally.
5. Remove from heat and use an immersion blender to blend the soup until smooth.
6. Stir in fresh cilantro.
7. Serve warm.

**Nutrition Info per Serving**

- Calories: 250
- Protein: 3g
- Carbohydrates: 25g
- Fiber: 6g
- Sugars: 8g
- Fat: 18g
- Saturated Fat: 10g
- Sodium: 180mg

**Servings: 4**
**Cooking Time: 30 minutes**

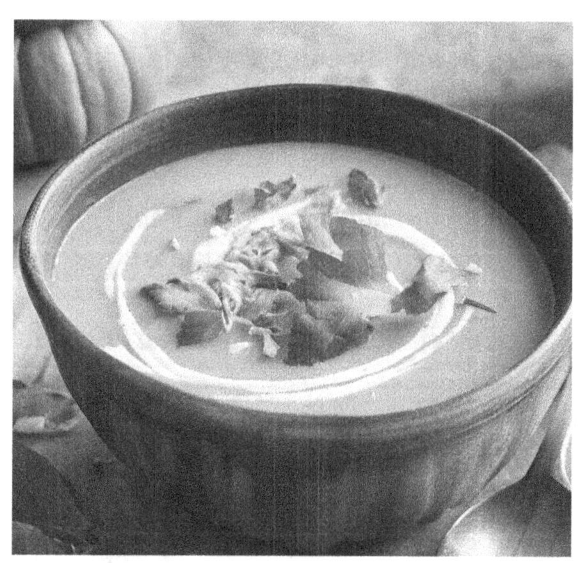

## 15. Cabbage and Potato Stew

**Ingredients**

- 2 tablespoons olive oil
- 1 onion, diced
- 3 garlic cloves, minced
- 4 cups green cabbage, chopped
- 3 potatoes, peeled and diced
- 4 cups low-sodium vegetable broth
- 1 teaspoon dried thyme
- 1/4 teaspoon ground black pepper
- 1 bay leaf
- 1 tablespoon apple cider vinegar
- 1 tablespoon fresh dill, chopped

**Instructions**

1. Heat olive oil in a large pot over medium heat.
2. Add diced onion and minced garlic. Sauté for 3-4 minutes until the onion is translucent.
3. Add chopped cabbage and diced potatoes. Cook for 5-7 minutes until the vegetables are slightly tender.
4. Stir in vegetable broth, dried thyme, ground black pepper, and bay leaf. Bring to a boil.
5. Reduce heat and simmer for 25-30 minutes until the vegetables are tender.
6. Remove the bay leaf and stir in apple cider vinegar.
7. Remove from heat and stir in fresh dill.
8. Serve warm.

**Nutrition Info per Serving**

- Calories: 200
- Protein: 5g
- Carbohydrates: 35g
- Fiber: 7g
- Sugars: 6g
- Fat: 6g
- Saturated Fat: 1g
- Sodium: 180mg

**Servings: 4**
**Cooking Time: 40 minutes**

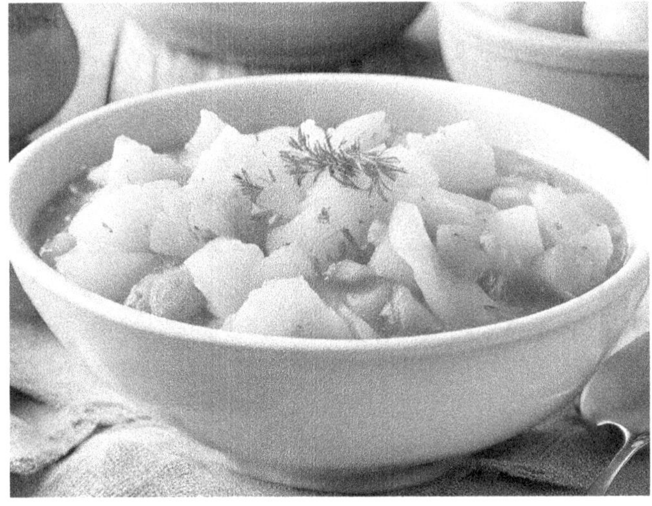

**16. Turkey and Kale Soup**
**Ingredients**

- 1 pound ground turkey
- 2 tablespoons olive oil
- 1 onion, diced
- 2 garlic cloves, minced
- 3 carrots, sliced
- 2 celery stalks, sliced
- 4 cups chopped kale, stems removed
- 6 cups low-sodium chicken broth
- 1 teaspoon dried thyme
- 1/4 teaspoon ground black pepper
- 1 tablespoon fresh parsley, chopped

**Instructions**

1. Heat olive oil in a large pot over medium heat.
2. Add ground turkey and cook until browned, about 5-7 minutes.
3. Add diced onion and minced garlic. Sauté for 3-4 minutes until the onion is translucent.
4. Add sliced carrots and celery. Cook for 5-7 minutes until the vegetables are slightly tender.
5. Stir in chopped kale, chicken broth, dried thyme, and ground black pepper. Bring to a boil.
6. Reduce heat and simmer for 25-30 minutes until the vegetables are tender.
7. Remove from heat and stir in fresh parsley.
8. Serve warm.

**Nutrition Info per Serving**

- Calories: 250
- Protein: 25g
- Carbohydrates: 15g
- Fiber: 4g
- Sugars: 6g
- Fat: 10g
- Saturated Fat: 2g
- Sodium: 200mg

**Servings: 4**
**Cooking Time: 45 minutes**

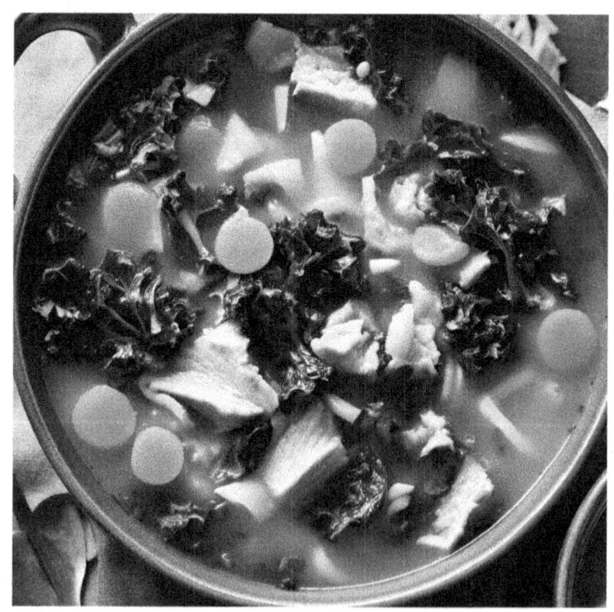

## 17. Spicy Black Bean Soup

### Ingredients

- 2 tablespoons olive oil
- 1 onion, diced
- 3 garlic cloves, minced
- 1 red bell pepper, diced
- 2 cans (15 ounces each) black beans, drained and rinsed
- 4 cups low-sodium vegetable broth
- 1 teaspoon ground cumin
- 1 teaspoon smoked paprika
- 1/4 teaspoon ground black pepper
- 1/4 teaspoon cayenne pepper
- 1 cup corn kernels (fresh or frozen)
- 1 lime, juiced
- 1/4 cup fresh cilantro, chopped

### Instructions

1. Heat olive oil in a large pot over medium heat.
2. Add diced onion and minced garlic. Sauté for 3-4 minutes until the onion is translucent.
3. Add diced red bell pepper and cook for 5-7 minutes until tender.
4. Stir in black beans, vegetable broth, ground cumin, smoked paprika, ground black pepper, and cayenne pepper. Bring to a boil.
5. Reduce heat and simmer for 20 minutes.
6. Stir in corn kernels and cook for an additional 5 minutes.
7. Remove from heat and stir in lime juice and fresh cilantro.
8. Serve warm.

### Nutrition Info per Serving

- Calories: 220
- Protein: 8g
- Carbohydrates: 35g
- Fiber: 10g
- Sugars: 4g
- Fat: 8g
- Saturated Fat: 1g
- Sodium: 180mg

**Servings: 4**
**Cooking Time: 30 minutes**

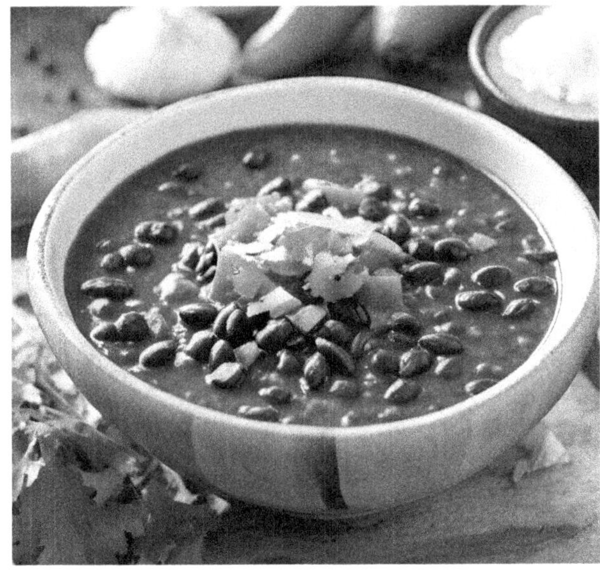

## 18. Cod and Parsnip Chowder

**Ingredients**

- 2 tablespoons olive oil
- 1 onion, diced
- 2 garlic cloves, minced
- 3 parsnips, peeled and diced
- 2 cups corn kernels (fresh or frozen)
- 4 cups low-sodium fish or vegetable broth
- 1 cup unsweetened almond milk
- 1 teaspoon dried thyme
- 1/4 teaspoon ground black pepper
- 1 pound cod fillets, cut into chunks
- 1 tablespoon fresh dill, chopped

**Instructions**

1. Heat olive oil in a large pot over medium heat.
2. Add diced onion and minced garlic. Sauté for 3-4 minutes until the onion is translucent.
3. Add diced parsnips and cook for 5-7 minutes until slightly tender.
4. Stir in corn kernels, fish or vegetable broth, almond milk, dried thyme, and ground black pepper. Bring to a boil.
5. Reduce heat and simmer for 20 minutes until the parsnips are tender.
6. Add cod chunks and cook for an additional 5-7 minutes until the fish is opaque and cooked through.
7. Remove from heat and stir in fresh dill.
8. Serve warm.

**Nutrition Info per Serving**

- Calories: 250
- Protein: 25g
- Carbohydrates: 25g
- Fiber: 5g
- Sugars: 8g
- Fat: 10g
- Saturated Fat: 1.5g
- Sodium: 200mg

**Servings: 4**

**Cooking Time: 40 minutes**

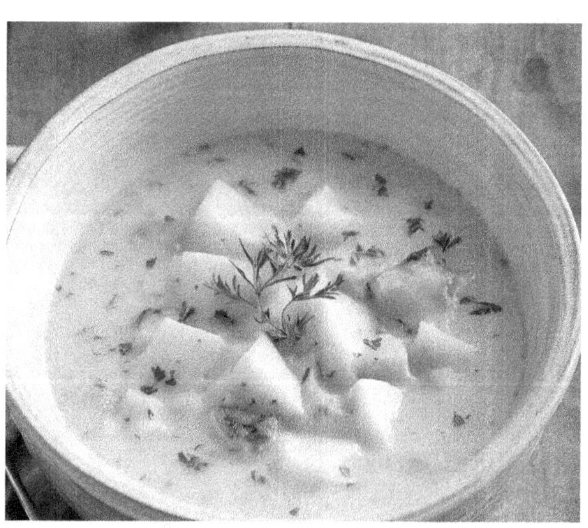

# 10-WEEK MEAL PLAN

## Week 1
Monday
- Breakfast: Green Goddess Smoothie
- Lunch: Vegetable Stuffed Portobello Mushrooms
- Dinner: Hearty Turkey and Vegetable Stew

Tuesday
- Breakfast: Turmeric Pineapple Smoothie
- Lunch: Spicy Kale and Coconut Stir Fry
- Dinner: Moroccan Vegetable Stew with Chickpeas

Wednesday
- Breakfast: Apple Cinnamon Porridge
- Lunch: Roasted Brussels Sprouts with Garlic and a side of quinoa
- Dinner: Fish Soup with Tomatoes and Herbs

Thursday
- Breakfast: Savory Oatmeal
- Lunch: Avocado and Tomato Salad
- Dinner: Chicken and Rice Soup with Lemon

Friday
- Breakfast: Scrambled Eggs with Spinach
- Lunch: Zucchini Noodles with Pesto
- Dinner: Lentil and Spinach Soup

Saturday
- Breakfast: Omelet with Mixed Veggies
- Lunch: Stuffed Bell Peppers with Quinoa
- Dinner: Beef Stew with Root Vegetables

Sunday
- Breakfast: Tofu Scramble
- Lunch: Spaghetti Squash with Tomato Sauce
- Dinner: Shrimp and Corn Chowder

## Week 2
Monday
- Breakfast: Egg Muffins
- Lunch: Broccoli and Garlic Sauté with brown rice
- Dinner: White Bean and Escarole Soup

Tuesday
- Breakfast: Ricotta and Berry Toast
- Lunch: Sweet Corn and Zucchini Pie
- Dinner: Turkey and Kale Soup

Wednesday
- Breakfast: Tahini and Honey Toast
- Lunch: Warm Quinoa and Roasted Vegetable Salad
- Dinner: Cod and Parsnip Chowder

Thursday
- Breakfast: Blueberry Oat Pancakes
- Lunch: Cabbage and Potato Stew
- Dinner: Vegan Mushroom and Tarragon Soup

Friday
- Breakfast: Cottage Cheese Pancakes
- Lunch: Stir-Fried Green Beans with Ginger
- Dinner: Italian Wedding Soup with Turkey Meatballs

Saturday
- Breakfast: Almond Flour Waffles
- Lunch: Cauliflower Steak with Turmeric and Cumin
- Dinner: Pumpkin and Coconut Milk Soup

Sunday
- Breakfast: Breakfast Quinoa Bowl
- Lunch: Vegetarian Stew with Barley and Winter Squash
- Dinner: Spicy Black Bean Soup

## Week 3

Monday
- Breakfast: Sweet Potato Hash
- Lunch: Roasted Turnips with Maple and Mustard
- Dinner: Baked Lemon Sole with Capers

Tuesday
- Breakfast: Buckwheat Porridge
- Lunch: Avocado and Tomato Salad
- Dinner: Barley and Mushroom Stew

Wednesday
- Breakfast: Muesli and Yogurt
- Lunch: Roasted Brussels Sprouts with Garlic
- Dinner: Shrimp and Corn Chowder

Thursday
- Breakfast: Berry and Flaxseed Yogurt
- Lunch: Spinach and Mushroom Frittata
- Dinner: Moroccan Vegetable Stew with Chickpeas

Friday
- Breakfast: Pear and Walnut Salad
- Lunch: Sweet Corn and Zucchini Pie
- Dinner: Turkey and Kale Soup

Saturday
- Breakfast: Peach Smoothie Bowl
- Lunch: Stuffed Bell Peppers with Quinoa
- Dinner: Hearty Turkey and Vegetable Stew

Sunday
- Breakfast: Scrambled Eggs with Spinach
- Lunch: Warm Quinoa and Roasted Vegetable Salad
- Dinner: Fish Soup with Tomatoes and Herbs

## Week 4

Monday
- Breakfast: Green Goddess Smoothie
- Lunch: Broccoli and Garlic Sauté with brown rice
- Dinner: Lentil and Spinach Soup

Tuesday
- Breakfast: Turmeric Pineapple Smoothie
- Lunch: Spaghetti Squash with Tomato Sauce
- Dinner: Chicken and Rice Soup with Lemon

Wednesday
- Breakfast: Apple Cinnamon Porridge
- Lunch: Cauliflower Steak with Turmeric and Cumin
- Dinner: Beef Stew with Root Vegetables

Thursday
- Breakfast: Savory Oatmeal
- Lunch: Zucchini Noodles with Pesto
- Dinner: Vegan Mushroom and Tarragon Soup

Friday
- Breakfast: Omelet with Mixed Veggies
- Lunch: Roasted Turnips with Maple and Mustard
- Dinner: Cod and Parsnip Chowder

Saturday
- Breakfast: Tofu Scramble
- Lunch: Sweet Corn and Zucchini Pie
- Dinner: Pumpkin and Coconut Milk Soup

Sunday
- Breakfast: Egg Muffins
- Lunch: Stuffed Bell Peppers with Quinoa
- Dinner: Italian Wedding Soup with Turkey Meatballs

## Week 5

Monday
- Breakfast: Ricotta and Berry Toast
- Lunch: Avocado and Tomato Salad
- Dinner: White Bean and Escarole Soup

Tuesday
- Breakfast: Tahini and Honey Toast
- Lunch: Roasted Brussels Sprouts with Garlic and a side of quinoa
- Dinner: Turkey and Kale Soup

Wednesday
- Breakfast: Blueberry Oat Pancakes
- Lunch: Spinach and Mushroom Frittata
- Dinner: Spicy Black Bean Soup

Thursday
- Breakfast: Cottage Cheese Pancakes
- Lunch: Stir-Fried Green Beans with Ginger
- Dinner: Moroccan Vegetable Stew with Chickpeas

Friday
- Breakfast: Almond Flour Waffles
- Lunch: Warm Quinoa and Roasted Vegetable Salad
- Dinner: Barley and Mushroom Stew

Saturday
- Breakfast: Breakfast Quinoa Bowl
- Lunch: Cauliflower Steak with Turmeric and Cumin
- Dinner: Hearty Turkey and Vegetable Stew

Sunday
- Breakfast: Sweet Potato Hash
- Lunch: Vegetarian Stew with Barley and Winter Squash
- Dinner: Shrimp and Corn Chowder

## Week 6

Monday
- Breakfast: Turmeric Pineapple Smoothie
- Lunch: Sweet Corn and Zucchini Pie
- Dinner: Spicy Black Bean Soup

Tuesday
- Breakfast: Apple Cinnamon Porridge
- Lunch: Zucchini Noodles with Pesto
- Dinner: Beef Stew with Root Vegetables

Wednesday
- Breakfast: Savory Oatmeal
- Lunch: Cauliflower Steak with Turmeric and Cumin
- Dinner: Moroccan Vegetable Stew with Chickpeas

Thursday
- Breakfast: Omelet with Mixed Veggies
- Lunch: Stir-Fried Green Beans with Ginger
- Dinner: Turkey and Kale Soup

Friday
- Breakfast: Tofu Scramble
- Lunch: Warm Quinoa and Roasted Vegetable Salad
- Dinner: Vegan Mushroom and Tarragon Soup

Saturday
- Breakfast: Egg Muffins
- Lunch: Avocado and Tomato Salad
- Dinner: Pumpkin and Coconut Milk Soup

Sunday
- Breakfast: Ricotta and Berry Toast
- Lunch: Stuffed Bell Peppers with Quinoa
- Dinner: Italian Wedding Soup with Turkey Meatballs

## Week 7

Monday
- Breakfast: Tahini and Honey Toast
- Lunch: Sweet Corn and Zucchini Pie
- Dinner: Cod and Parsnip Chowder

Tuesday
- Breakfast: Blueberry Oat Pancakes
- Lunch: Spinach and Mushroom Frittata
- Dinner: Hearty Turkey and Vegetable Stew

Wednesday
- Breakfast: Cottage Cheese Pancakes
- Lunch: Stir-Fried Green Beans with Ginger
- Dinner: Spicy Black Bean Soup

Thursday
- Breakfast: Almond Flour Waffles
- Lunch: Warm Quinoa and Roasted Vegetable Salad
- Dinner: Beef Stew with Root Vegetables

Friday
- Breakfast: Breakfast Quinoa Bowl
- Lunch: Cauliflower Steak with Turmeric and Cumin
- Dinner: Moroccan Vegetable Stew with Chickpeas

Saturday

- Breakfast: Sweet Potato Hash
- Lunch: Zucchini Noodles with Pesto
- Dinner: Vegan Mushroom and Tarragon Soup

Sunday

- Breakfast: Buckwheat Porridge
- Lunch: Roasted Brussels Sprouts with Garlic and a side of quinoa
- Dinner: Chicken and Rice Soup with Lemon

## Week 8

Monday

- Breakfast: Muesli and Yogurt
- Lunch: Avocado and Tomato Salad
- Dinner: White Bean and Escarole Soup

Tuesday

- Breakfast: Berry and Flaxseed Yogurt
- Lunch: Stir-Fried Green Beans with Ginger
- Dinner: Turkey and Kale Soup

Wednesday

- Breakfast: Pear and Walnut Salad
- Lunch: Sweet Corn and Zucchini Pie
- Dinner: Spicy Black Bean Soup

Thursday

- Breakfast: Peach Smoothie Bowl
- Lunch: Spinach and Mushroom Frittata
- Dinner: Cod and Parsnip Chowder

Friday

- Breakfast: Scrambled Eggs with Spinach
- Lunch: Warm Quinoa and Roasted Vegetable Salad
- Dinner: Pumpkin and Coconut Milk Soup

Saturday

- Breakfast: Omelet with Mixed Veggies
- Lunch: Avocado and Tomato Salad
- Dinner: Italian Wedding Soup with Turkey Meatballs

Sunday

- Breakfast: Tofu Scramble
- Lunch: Cauliflower Steak with Turmeric and Cumin
- Dinner: Hearty Turkey and Vegetable Stew

## Week 9

Monday
- Breakfast: Egg Muffins
- Lunch: Sweet Corn and Zucchini Pie
- Dinner: Vegan Mushroom and Tarragon Soup

Tuesday
- Breakfast: Ricotta and Berry Toast
- Lunch: Zucchini Noodles with Pesto
- Dinner: Beef Stew with Root Vegetables

Wednesday
- Breakfast: Tahini and Honey Toast
- Lunch: Stir-Fried Green Beans with Ginger
- Dinner: Moroccan Vegetable Stew with Chickpeas

Thursday
- Breakfast: Blueberry Oat Pancakes
- Lunch: Spinach and Mushroom Frittata
- Dinner: Turkey and Kale Soup

Friday
- Breakfast: Cottage Cheese Pancakes
- Lunch: Warm Quinoa and Roasted Vegetable Salad
- Dinner: Spicy Black Bean Soup

Saturday
- Breakfast: Almond Flour Waffles
- Lunch: Cauliflower Steak with Turmeric and Cumin
- Dinner: Pumpkin and Coconut Milk Soup

Sunday
- Breakfast: Breakfast Quinoa Bowl
- Lunch: Avocado and Tomato Salad
- Dinner: Italian Wedding Soup with Turkey Meatballs

## Week 10

Monday
- Breakfast: Sweet Potato Hash
- Lunch: Stir-Fried Green Beans with Ginger
- Dinner: Cod and Parsnip Chowder

Tuesday
- Breakfast: Buckwheat Porridge
- Lunch: Spinach and Mushroom Frittata
- Dinner: Hearty Turkey and Vegetable Stew

Wednesday
- Breakfast: Muesli and Yogurt
- Lunch: Warm Quinoa and Roasted Vegetable Salad
- Dinner: Moroccan Vegetable Stew with Chickpeas

Thursday
- Breakfast: Berry and Flaxseed Yogurt
- Lunch: Cauliflower Steak with Turmeric and Cumin
- Dinner: Vegan Mushroom and Tarragon Soup

Friday
- Breakfast: Pear and Walnut Salad
- Lunch: Sweet Corn and Zucchini Pie
- Dinner: Turkey and Kale Soup

Saturday
- Breakfast: Peach Smoothie Bowl
- Lunch: Zucchini Noodles with Pesto
- Dinner: Spicy Black Bean Soup

Sunday
- Breakfast: Scrambled Eggs with Spinach
- Lunch: Avocado and Tomato Salad
- Dinner: Pumpkin and Coconut Milk Soup

# Weekly Meal planner+ Journal

|  | BREAKFAST | LUNCH | DINNER | SNACKS |
|---|---|---|---|---|
| MON |  |  |  |  |
| TUE |  |  |  |  |
| WED |  |  |  |  |
| THU |  |  |  |  |
| FRI |  |  |  |  |
| SAT |  |  |  |  |
| SUN |  |  |  |  |

How did you feel when you were first diagnosed with autoimmune hepatitis, and what concerns do you have about starting a new diet?

# Weekly Meal planner+ Journal

| | BREAKFAST | LUNCH | DINNER | SNACKS |
|---|---|---|---|---|
| MON | | | | |
| TUE | | | | |
| WED | | | | |
| THU | | | | |
| FRI | | | | |
| SAT | | | | |
| SUN | | | | |

**Describe your current eating habits. Which foods do you eat regularly, and which ones do you think might need to change to better manage your condition?**

........................................................................................................

........................................................................................................

........................................................................................................

........................................................................................................

........................................................................................................

........................................................................................................

# Weekly Meal planner+ Journal

| | BREAKFAST | LUNCH | DINNER | SNACKS |
|---|---|---|---|---|
| MON | | | | |
| TUE | | | | |
| WED | | | | |
| THU | | | | |
| FRI | | | | |
| SAT | | | | |
| SUN | | | | |

What symptoms of autoimmune hepatitis do you experience most frequently, and how do you think your diet might be impacting these symptoms?

# Weekly Meal planner+ Journal

| | BREAKFAST | LUNCH | DINNER | SNACKS |
|---|---|---|---|---|
| MON | | | | |
| TUE | | | | |
| WED | | | | |
| THU | | | | |
| FRI | | | | |
| SAT | | | | |
| SUN | | | | |

**What do you already know about the autoimmune hepatitis diet, and what areas are you most eager to learn more about?**

.................................................................................................................

.................................................................................................................

.................................................................................................................

.................................................................................................................

.................................................................................................................

.................................................................................................................

# Weekly Meal planner + Journal

| | BREAKFAST | LUNCH | DINNER | SNACKS |
|---|---|---|---|---|
| MON | | | | |
| TUE | | | | |
| WED | | | | |
| THU | | | | |
| FRI | | | | |
| SAT | | | | |
| SUN | | | | |

How do you currently plan your grocery shopping, and what changes might you need to make to ensure you buy foods that support your health?

........................................................................................................

........................................................................................................

........................................................................................................

........................................................................................................

........................................................................................................

........................................................................................................

# Weekly Meal planner+ Journal

| | BREAKFAST | LUNCH | DINNER | SNACKS |
|---|---|---|---|---|
| MON | | | | |
| TUE | | | | |
| WED | | | | |
| THU | | | | |
| FRI | | | | |
| SAT | | | | |
| SUN | | | | |

How comfortable are you with cooking and preparing meals? What challenges do you foresee in preparing meals that fit the autoimmune hepatitis diet?

......................................................................................................

......................................................................................................

......................................................................................................

......................................................................................................

......................................................................................................

......................................................................................................

# Weekly Meal planner+ Journal

|  | BREAKFAST | LUNCH | DINNER | SNACKS |
|---|---|---|---|---|
| MON |  |  |  |  |
| TUE |  |  |  |  |
| WED |  |  |  |  |
| THU |  |  |  |  |
| FRI |  |  |  |  |
| SAT |  |  |  |  |
| SUN |  |  |  |  |

Who in your life can support you as you start this new diet? How can they help you stay motivated and on track?

........................................................................................................

........................................................................................................

........................................................................................................

........................................................................................................

........................................................................................................

........................................................................................................

# Weekly Meal planner+ Journal

|  | BREAKFAST | LUNCH | DINNER | SNACKS |
|---|---|---|---|---|
| MON |  |  |  |  |
| TUE |  |  |  |  |
| WED |  |  |  |  |
| THU |  |  |  |  |
| FRI |  |  |  |  |
| SAT |  |  |  |  |
| SUN |  |  |  |  |

How often do you eat out at restaurants, and what strategies can you use to make healthier choices when dining out?

# Weekly Meal planner+ Journal

| | BREAKFAST | LUNCH | DINNER | SNACKS |
|---|---|---|---|---|
| MON | | | | |
| TUE | | | | |
| WED | | | | |
| THU | | | | |
| FRI | | | | |
| SAT | | | | |
| SUN | | | | |

What are your specific goals for following the autoimmune hepatitis diet? Consider both short-term and long-term objectives.

# Weekly Meal planner + Journal

| | BREAKFAST | LUNCH | DINNER | SNACKS |
|---|---|---|---|---|
| MON | | | | |
| TUE | | | | |
| WED | | | | |
| THU | | | | |
| FRI | | | | |
| SAT | | | | |
| SUN | | | | |

What potential barriers do you anticipate in following the autoimmune hepatitis diet, and how can you plan to overcome them?

# Weekly Meal planner+ Journal

| | BREAKFAST | LUNCH | DINNER | SNACKS |
| --- | --- | --- | --- | --- |
| MON | | | | |
| TUE | | | | |
| WED | | | | |
| THU | | | | |
| FRI | | | | |
| SAT | | | | |
| SUN | | | | |

Are there any specific cooking skills or techniques you would like to learn or improve to help you follow the diet more effectively?

# Weekly Meal planner+ Journal

| | BREAKFAST | LUNCH | DINNER | SNACKS |
|---|---|---|---|---|
| MON | | | | |
| TUE | | | | |
| WED | | | | |
| THU | | | | |
| FRI | | | | |
| SAT | | | | |
| SUN | | | | |

How do your emotions influence your eating habits, and what strategies can you use to manage emotional eating while following the diet?

# Scan the QR code below to get a surprise bonus

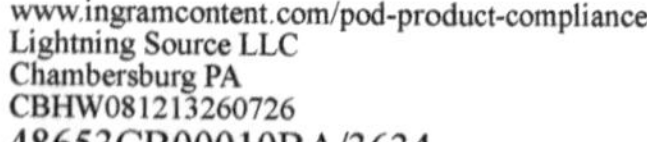